A Divine Wellness Journey

A 28-DAY JOURNAL TO UNLEASH THE MOST POWERFUL YOU

Live Beautifully. Feel Divine

A Divine Wellness Journey is a 28-day reset for the woman ready to reclaim her power, nourish her body & reconnect with herself. Inside you will find simple smoothie recipes, empowering affirmations, and reflective journal prompts -- all design to help you unleash the most powerful version of yourself. Own your evolution.

Tarsha Whitaker Calloway

Divine Original logo design: Clark K. Calloway

Published in the United States by

BLUE TREE PRESS
The root of life begins with a good book

Visit our website at www.bluetreepress.com

Printed in the United States
First Printing September 2025
ISBN: 979-8-218-69140-0

Calloway, Tarsha Whitaker
A wellness journal for good health and divine inspiration

Important Health Disclaimer: A Divine Wellness Journey is intended solely for informational and educational purposes and not as medical counseling. Please consult a medical or healthcare professional if you have questions about any health conditions.

Additionally, the recipes feature a variety of ingredients, including nuts and grains. If you have food allergies, please carefully read each recipe to determine if it is safe for you to consume.

The publisher and author are not responsible for any adverse effects or consequences resulting from the use of any of the suggestions or preparations discussed in this book.

Table of *Contents*

Drink Beautifully. Feel Divine

Dedication

To my husband—
Your unwavering support, gentle strength, and belief in every version of me have carried me through more than words can ever fully express. Thank you for loving all of who I am and holding space for who I continue to become.

To my son—
You are the brightest light in my life. The smartest, most incredible son a mother could be blessed to have. Watching you grow is one of my greatest joys. I love you beyond the moon and back, always.

To my mother—
You are the epitome of motherhood. Your grace, your prayers, your sacrifices, and your endless love continue to guide me. You taught me how to give, how to rise, and how to mother with heart.

To my college roommate and dearest friend—
You are more than a friend—you are a soul sister and one of my loudest, proudest cheerleaders. Your encouragement, laughter, and love have meant the world to me.

To my family and friends—
Thank you for showing up for me—even when it wasn't easy, even when it wasn't convenient. I see you. I honor you. And I carry your love with me on every page of this journey.

This book is a piece of my heart. And to everyone who has poured into me, lifted me up, prayed for me, laughed with me, or stood beside me—please know that **I appreciate you more than I could ever say; thank you.**

The Heart Behind the Journey.

The Sacred Shift.

As a philanthropic leader, businesswoman, mentor, wife, and mother—I spent decades nurturing others, building legacies, and pouring into people, purpose, and progress. From boardrooms to fundraisers, from home to community, I have shown up with strength, strategy, and heart.

But something shifted.

Not in the demands of the world—but within. A quiet knowing emerged: it was time to pour inward. Time to reclaim the energy once freely given. Time to prioritize self in a way that felt both bold and gentle.

I no longer wanted to hustle through healing. I wanted presence. Lightness. Space.

This journal is the sacred expression of that shift.

A Divine Wellness Journey is more than a collection of smoothie recipes. It's a 28-day wellness guide designed to help women reclaim, reset, and realign. It offers nourishment for the body, affirmations for the spirit, and journaling prompts to reconnect with purpose.

Created for women who lead, give, love, mentor, and do it all—this journey is for those who are finally ready to do something deeply meaningful for themselves.

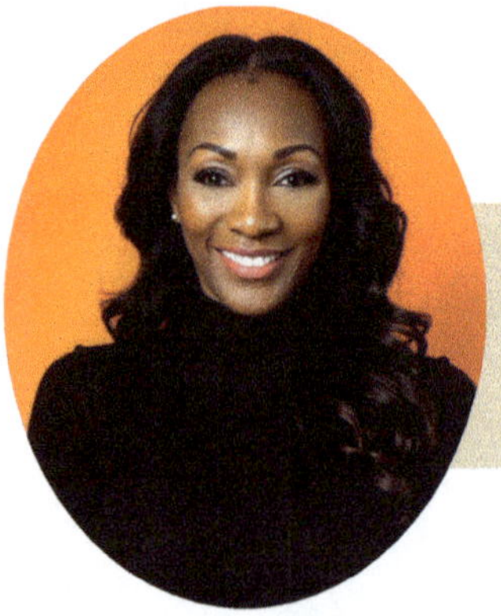

It's for the busy woman entering a new chapter.
For the mother navigating hormonal shifts with grace.
For the entrepreneur who needs to soften the edges of her ambition.

For the nurturer who's ready to be nurtured.
Each page encourages intention—blending together daily smoothies, mindful reflection, and emotional release. No pressure. No perfection.

Just a reminder:

It's your turn.
Your turn to feel whole.
Your turn to rest and replenish.
Your turn to glow, inside and out.
Let this journal be a mirror, a reset, a refuge.
You are a divine original—brilliant, becoming, and beautifully designed to bloom in your own time.

Live Beautifully. Feel Divine

This is the moment we return to ourselves—you have poured into others with purpose now pour into yourself with power One sip one step one sacred pause at a time Let the journey begin

— Tarsha W. Calloway

Best Times *to Blend*

- Start on Monday morning. Sunday night prep and shopping
- Morning: Lemon Ginger Shot on an empty stomach (daily)
- Breakfast Smoothie (nourishing + energizing)
- Afternoon/Evening Smoothie (relax, hydrating & cleansing)

Shop + Prep with Intention

Each week for the next four weeks, you'll carve out a little time to shop and prep for your smoothies. This is your moment to set yourself up for ease, simplicity, and success.

If you plan to enjoy your smoothies for both breakfast and lunch, blend them both in the morning. Pour one into your favorite glass or tumbler to take with you. It's that easy—and yes, you're still nourishing yourself beautifully on the go.

This isn't about being perfect. It's about being prepared.

Your blender, your greens, your sacred pause—that's your wellness ritual now.

Replace 2 Meals a Day *with Love*

Each day, you'll replace two meals with the smoothies outlined in your plan. You can enjoy:

- Two nourishing smoothies
- One healthy, solid food meal
- Up to two light snacks if needed (like fruit, nuts, or veggies)

I gently recommend replacing breakfast and dinner, giving your body a reset in the morning and a light, easy close at night. But if your rhythm calls for breakfast and lunch, honor what works best for you. This journey is here to meet you where you are.

Remember: This is about fueling your body and your spirit—not restriction, but restoration.

Because flexibility is a part of wellness.

One of the most empowering parts of this journey is knowing that it doesn't have to be rigid. Life isn't, and your smoothies shouldn't be either.

There may be moments when you're missing an ingredient, want to adjust for taste, or need to work with what's already in your kitchen. The beauty of smoothies is that they welcome flexibility.

Here are a few helpful guidelines and gentle swaps to keep your experience stress-free, nourishing, and delicious.

Greens: Switch It Up

with Confidence

You can use any leafy green in these recipes. The only invitation I extend is this: rotate them. Your body will thank you for the variety.

Some greens are milder (and more beginner-friendly), while others are bold and assertive:

- Spinach – Soft, mellow, easy to blend.
- Kale – Earthier flavor, pairs beautifully with citrus.
- Arugula – Peppery and strong. A little goes a long way.

Pre-washed mixes, such as Power Greens, are a great option—they combine several varieties, making it effortless to rotate through different greens.

Tip: Avoid using the same greens for more than two consecutive days. A simple switch can keep your nutrients diverse, and your taste buds satisfied.

Fruit Swaps *Made Simple*

Smoothies are forgiving. When one fruit is out of reach, there's almost always another that steps in with ease. Here's a quick substitution guide:

Original	Swap With...
Banana	Avocado (creamy, less sweet)
Oranges	Clementines, Tangerines
Pineapple	Oranges, Mangoes, Peaches
Pear	Apples, Peaches, Plums
Melon	Any other melon (Cantaloupe, Honeydew, Watermelon)
Mango	Papaya, Peaches

Each of these alternatives keeps your smoothie vibrant and aligned with your wellness goals.

This is your journey. And it gets to feel good.

Liquid & Nut Butter Substitutions

Your base liquid plays a key role in texture and taste. Feel free to alternate based on what you prefer or have on hand:

Almond Milk ↔ Coconut Milk

Both offer a creamy, neutral base perfect for most blends.

Coconut Water ↔ Filtered Water

Coconut water adds natural sweetness and electrolytes, but regular water works in a pinch—it just softens the flavor a bit.

Nut Butters

Peanut butter, almond butter, and cashew butter are all interchangeable. Each offers healthy fats and protein—choose the option that suits your taste and dietary needs.

There's no single "right way" to do this. Every blend is a chance to honor your body and make a loving choice—for where you are right now.

Swap what you need. Adjust what you want.

Stay rooted in grace and know that every sip is part of your return to yourself.

This journey is about embracing transformation discovering inner strength and celebrating a healthier more vibrant you

It's not about weight loss.

While you may experience weight release as your body resets and restores, the true purpose of this program is deeper than a number on the scale. A Divine Wellness Journey is about reclaiming yourself—physically, emotionally, spiritually, and energetically.

- This is a moment to return to you.
- To slow down.
- To prep with intention.
- To blend with love.
- To sip with presence.

Each smoothie, each affirmation, and each pause is an invitation to reconnect with the divine original that you are. This journey is about honoring your body, restoring your rhythm, and prioritizing your well-being.

You are not here to shrink. You are here to shine.
And most of all—remember, **it's your turn.**

Your Journal is Your Sacred Space

This is where the transformation deepens.

Journal whenever your heart desires. Whether it's a few lines in the morning or a soul-cleansing reflection at night, journaling is your invitation to come home to yourself.

This 28-day journey isn't just about smoothies—it's about self-reclamation. And the page is where that reclamation becomes real. This is your space to:

- Reflect on how you feel inside and out
- Witness your progress—physical, emotional, and spiritual
- Track the shifts happening in your body, your thoughts, and your energy
- Be radically honest, deeply gentle, and wholly you

> *You don't need perfect words.*
> *You just need presence.*
> *You don't need to hold back.*
> *You need a moment to be still.*

I will offer prompts to guide your reflections and affirmations to ground your truth. Use them—or let your spirit write its own. Just know this: every word is a form of wellness. Every pause you take to write is a reclamation of your time, your voice, your divine rhythm.

It's okay..

It's okay to take your time.
It's okay to feel everything.
It's okay to show up as you are.

This is your journey.
This is your healing.
And this... is your turn.

A gentle reminder that reclamation takes time, and you are enough every step of the way.

28 DAYS
AT-A GLANCE

Week 1:
RECLAIM + CLEANSE

I am a divine original, and today,
I reclaim every part of me
that I've neglected.
I honor my body by returning to
it with grace, presence, and care.

Week 1: Reclaim + Cleanse

This week is about returning to the center—clearing what no longer serves you, calming the gut, and reclaiming the vibrant energy that has been tucked beneath stress, sugar, and survival mode.

DAY 1
Reclaim Your Rhythm

Green Reset
Banana Calm

2 Healthy Snacks
1 Healthy Meal

DAY 2
Detox the Distractions

Berry Wake-Up
Cucumber Zen

2 Healthy Snacks
1 Healthy Meal

DAY 3
Breathe & Reset

Citrus Glow
Avocado Balance

2 Healthy Snacks
1 Healthy Meal

DAY 4
Calm the Gut

Gut Greens
Soothing Spice

2 Healthy Snacks
1 Healthy Meal

DAY 5
Flush the Fog

Energy Elixir
Root Revival

2 Healthy Snacks
1 Healthy Meal

DAY 6
Choose You Again

Pineapple Power
Hormone Helper

2 Healthy Snacks
1 Healthy Meal

DAY 7
Soft Reset

Sunrise Smoothie
Evening Ease

2 Healthy Snacks
1 Healthy Meal

> *I am not starting over—*
> *I am returning to myself.*
> *Everything I need has*
> *always been within me.*

Week 1 Grocery List:

Reclaim + Cleanse

PRODUCE

- 3 bananas
- 2 green apples
- 1 pear
- 2 oranges
- 1 lime
- 1 lemon
- 1 cup pineapple
- 1 cup mango
- 1 cup blueberries
- 1 papaya
- 2 medium carrots
- 1 small beet
- 1 avocado
- pumpkin purée
- fresh ginger
- fresh turmeric
- 1 small cucumber
- 2 stalks celery
- romaine lettuce
- mint leaves
- spinach
- cup kale

PANTRY / DRY GOODS

- Chia seeds
- Ground flaxseed
- Almond butter or nut butter of choice
- Cinnamon
- Nutmeg
- Vanilla extract
- Dates (3–5)

REFRIGERATED / NON-DAIRY

- Unsweetened almond milk (approx. 4–5 cups)
- Unsweetened oat milk (approx. 2–3 cups)
- Coconut water (approx. 4–5 cups)
- Aloe vera juice (unsweetened, optional)

“

Week 2: RECHARGE + NOURISH

I am a divine original, fully deserving of rest and renewal. My energy is sacred, and I choose to recharge from a place of love—not urgency.

”

Week 2: Recharge + Nourish

This week is all about restoring energy, uplifting mood, and rebuilding strength. You're refueling the body with nutrients that support immunity, hydration, circulation, and clarity.

DAY 8
Fuel Your Fire

Ginger Citrus Spark
Almond Energy

2 Healthy Snacks
1 Healthy Meal

DAY 9
Rise Gently

Watermelon Rise
Peach Recharge

2 Healthy Snacks
1 Healthy Meal

DAY 10
Feel the Flow

Beet Vitality
Coconut Calm

2 Healthy Snacks
1 Healthy Meal

DAY 11
Stay Steady

Apple Cider Glow
Mocha Mood

2 Healthy Snacks
1 Healthy Meal

DAY 12
Light Up Inside

Sunshine Blend
Lavender Lemon

2 Healthy Snacks
1 Healthy Meal

DAY 13
Strong & Soft

Berry Boost
Cucumber Aloe

2 Healthy Snacks
1 Healthy Meal

DAY 14
Recharge & Reflect

Golden Recharge
Lavender Dream

2 Healthy Snacks
1 Healthy Meal

> *"This is the week I protect my peace, nourish my energy, and power up from within."*

Week 2 Grocery List:

Recharge + Nourish

PRODUCE

- 3 bananas
- 1 green apple
- 2 oranges
- 1 lemon
- 1 lime
- 1 cup pineapple
- 1 cup mango
- 1 watermelon
- 1 cup peaches
- Spinach 1/2 avocado
- 1 beet
- 1 medium carrot
- 1 cucumber
- 1 pear
- 1-inch piece ginger
- Mint leaves
- Lavender (optional)
- Mixed berries

PANTRY / DRY GOODS

- Almond butter or nut butter
- Chia seeds
- Ground flaxseed
- Cinnamon
- Turmeric
- Cacao powder
- Dates (5–6)
- Honey
- Apple cider vinegar
- Vanilla extract

REFRIGERATED / NON-DAIRY

- Unsweetened almond milk (approx. 5 cups)
- Oat milk (approx. 4 cups)
- Coconut milk (approx. 1–2 cups)
- Cold brew coffee (optional)
- Aloe juice (optional)

Week 3: RESTORE + HYDRATE

I am a divine original, designed to heal and restore. I trust the wisdom within me to bring balance, peace, and harmony back to my body and spirit.

Week 3: Restore + Hydrate

This week is about replenishing from within—balancing hormones, improving sleep, soothing stress, and grounding yourself in nourishment that supports a calm, restored body.

DAY 15
Ground & Breath

Sweet Root Balance
Chamomile Calm

2 Healthy Snacks
1 Healthy Meal

DAY 16
Release & Reset

Hormone Harmony
Golden Sleep

2 Healthy Snacks
1 Healthy Meal

DAY 17
Nourish Deeply

Pear & Spinach Reset
Tahini Glow

2 Healthy Snacks
1 Healthy Meal

DAY 18
Root & Rebuild

Blueberry Boost
Warm Spice

2 Healthy Snacks
1 Healthy Meal

DAY 19
Restore Your Fire

Maca Monday
Coconut Lavender Ease

2 Healthy Snacks
1 Healthy Meal

DAY 20
Digest & Declutter

Papaya & Lime Digestive
Pear Vanilla Chai

2 Healthy Snacks
1 Healthy Meal

DAY 21
Rest & Reflect

Golden Greens
Evening Restore

2 Healthy Snacks
1 Healthy Meal

> *"I am allowed to rest, to reset, and to rise. My healing is valid, beautiful, and mine."*

Week 3 Grocery List:

Restore + Hydrate

PRODUCE

- 3 bananas
- 2 pears
- 1 apple
- 1 lime
- 1 lemon
- 1 cup papaya chunks
- 1 cup pineapple
- 1 cup blueberries
- 1 beet
- 1 medium carrot
- 1 cucumber
- Spinach (2 handfuls)
- Ginger (1-inch piece)
- Mint
- Pumpkin purée (1/2 cup)

PANTRY / DRY GOODS

- Chia seeds
- Ground flaxseed
- Maca powder
- Cacao powder
- Tahini
- Cinnamon
- Nutmeg
- Cardamom
- Vanilla extract
- Dates (5–7)

REFRIGERATED / NON-DAIRY

- Unsweetened almond milk (approx. 4–5 cups)
- Oat milk (approx. 4 cups)
- Coconut water (approx. 2–3 cups)
- Coconut milk (approx. 2 cups)
- Chamomile tea bags (for blending)
- Lavender (culinary-grade, optional)

Week 4:
RADIATE + GLOW

I am a divine original, and my light is undeniable. I radiate joy, beauty, and truth simply by choosing to show up for myself fully and unapologetically.

Week 4: Radiate + Glow

You've done the work to reclaim, recharge, and restore. Now it's time to radiate—through your skin, your energy, your presence, and your joy.

DAY 22
Glow From Within

Tropical Glow
Cacao Calm

2 Healthy Snacks
1 Healthy Meal

DAY 23
Radiant Strength

Berry Beauty
Golden Apple

2 Healthy Snacks
1 Healthy Meal

DAY 24
Step Into Shine

Strawberry Citrus Spark
Honey Almond Radiant

2 Healthy Snacks
1 Healthy Meal

DAY 25
Celebrate You

Sun-Kissed Carrot
Moon Milk Dream

2 Healthy Snacks
1 Healthy Meal

DAY 26
Own Your Glow

Papaya Power
Spice Berry Calm

2 Healthy Snacks
1 Healthy Meal

DAY 27
Radiate Ease

Melon Mint Hydrator
Warm Lavender Vanilla

2 Healthy Snacks
1 Healthy Meal

DAY 28
Shine On

Pineapple Citrus Blast
Divine Glow Elixir

2 Healthy Snacks
1 Healthy Meal

> *I no longer dim to fit in. This is my light, my turn, and my time to shine.*

Week 4 Grocery List:
Radiate + Glow

PRODUCE

- 3 bananas
- 1 green apple
- 1 orange
- 1 lemon
- 1 lime
- 1 cup pineapple
- 1 cup mango
- 1 cup strawberries
- 1 cup mixed berries
- 1 cup papaya
- 1 cup honeydew or cantaloupe
- 1 carrot
- 1 cucumber
- Spinach (1 handful)
- Mint leaves
- Ginger (1-inch piece)

PANTRY / DRY GOODS

- Chia seeds
- Ground flaxseed
- Cinnamon
- Nutmeg
- Cacao powder
- Vanilla extract
- Dates (4–5)
- Honey
- Ashwagandha (optional adaptogen)
- Lavender (culinary-safe, optional)

LIQUIDS

- Unsweetened almond milk (5 cups)
- Oat milk (3–4 cups)
- Coconut water (3–4 cups)

Daily Lemon Ginger Shot

RECIPE:

- 4 medium lemons
- 1 pound of fresh ginger
- 200 ml cold water
- Pinch of cayenne pepper
- 1 tablespoon of honey (optional)

Make it turmeric ginger shot by swapping half of the ginger for fresh turmeric, or add one teaspoon of ground turmeric before blending.

Gather the ingredients. Wash and dry the ginger, then coarsely chop. Slice the peels off the lemon and dice them; add to a blender. Add the ginger, lemon juice, water, and honey. Blend on high until a mostly smooth, thick mixture forms, stopping to scrape down the bowl occasionally, about 2 minutes. Transfer the mixture to a cheesecloth. Gather up the edges of the cloth and twist, squeezing the ginger pulp into a ball inside the cloth. Squeeze well and continue to twist until no more liquid is dripping out of the cloth and the pulp is dehydrated. Discard the pulp. Transfer the liquid into a bottle using a funnel and chill.

Benefits of Daily Ginger Shots: Daily ginger shots offer a range of potential benefits, including supporting digestive health, boosting immune function, and promoting circulation.

GUT HEALTH HIGHLIGHTS

- Add chia or flaxseed to smoothies for fiber and digestion
- Use ginger, lemon, and turmeric to reduce inflammation
- Choose leafy greens like kale, arugula, and spinach for diversity
- Drink plenty of water with fresh herbs or citrus slices
- Include prebiotic-rich foods like bananas, garlic, and oats

SMOOTHIE RECIPES

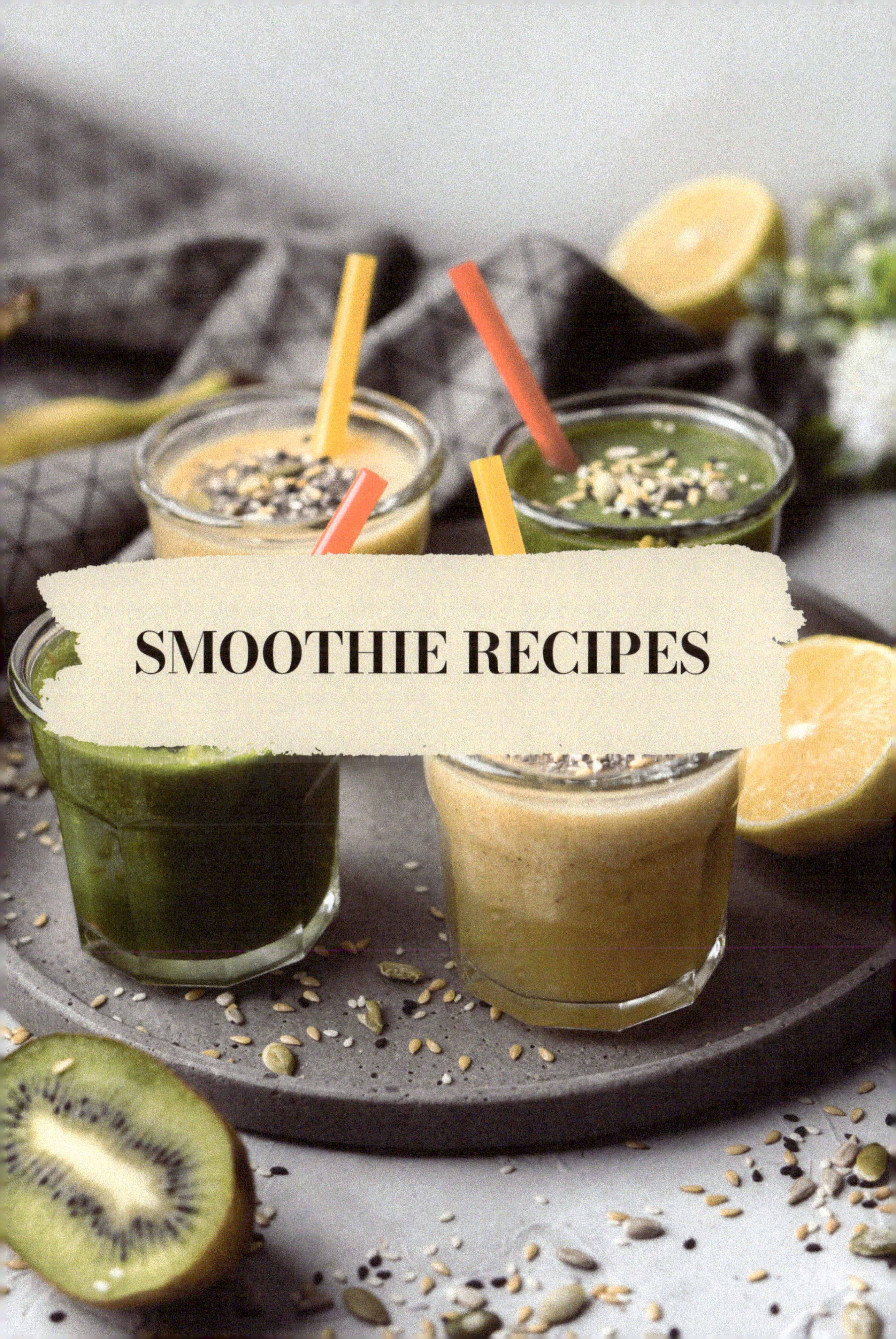

Day 1: Reclaim *Your Rhythm*

Every day is a new beginning. Take a deep breath, smile, and start again.

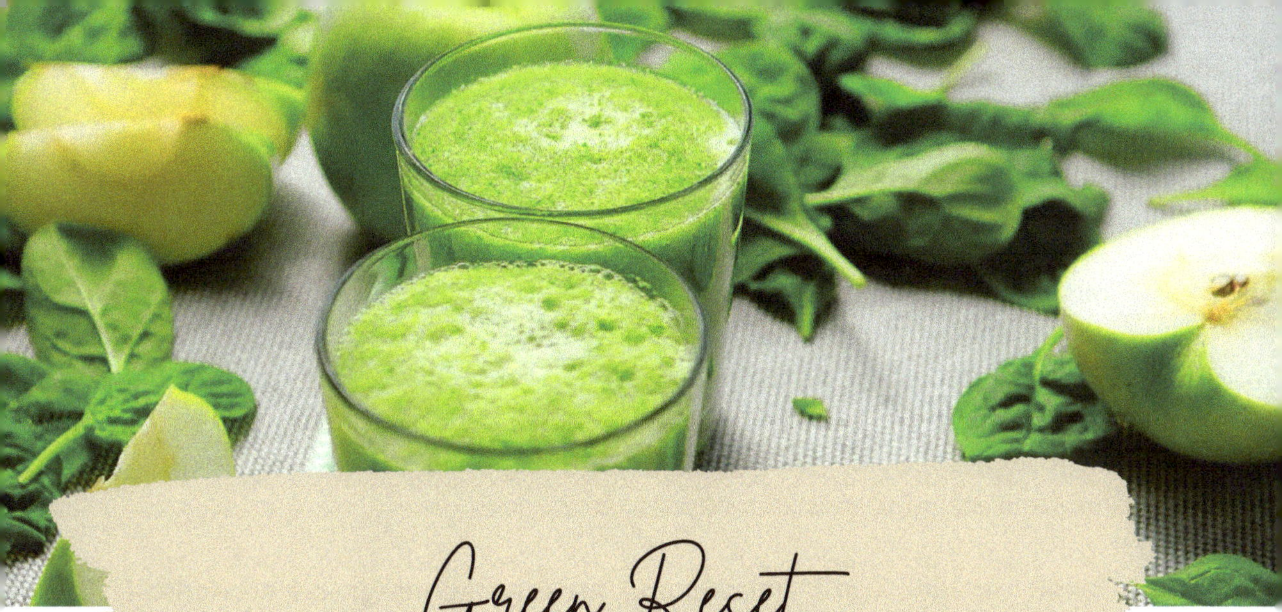

Green Reset

Spinach, cucumber, green apple, lemon, ginger, coconut water

This refreshing Green Reset Smoothie is packed with nutrients and is designed to promote hydration, support digestion, and aid in liver cleansing. Here's how to make it:

INGREDIENTS:

- 1 cup fresh spinach
- 1/2 medium cucumber
- 1 green
- Juice of 1 lemon
- 1-inch piece of fresh ginger
- 1 cup coconut water

OPTIONAL ADD-INS:

- 1 tablespoon chia seeds: For added fiber and omega-3 fatty acids.
- 1 tablespoon honey or maple syrup: For a sweeter taste.
- 1/2 ripe avocado: For creaminess and healthy fats.
- 1/2 cup ice cubes: To chill your smoothie and make it extra refreshing.

INSTRUCTIONS:

1. Rinse the spinach thoroughly under cold water to remove any dirt or grit. Peel the cucumber (if desired, for a milder taste) and chop it into smaller pieces. Core and chop the green apple into chunks, leaving the skin on for added nutrients. Peel the ginger and slice it thinly. Cut the lemon in half and juice it using a citrus juicer or a fork.

2. In a high-speed blender, add the fresh spinach, cucumber, green apple, lemon juice, ginger, and coconut water.

3. Blend on high until smooth and creamy, about 30-60 seconds. If the smoothie is too thick for your liking, you can always add more coconut water to reach your desired consistency.

4. Pour the smoothie into a glass or to-go bottle. If you've made enough, you can store leftovers in the fridge for up to 24 hours, but it's best enjoyed fresh.

TIPS:

- For the best flavor, use fresh, high-quality ingredients.

- Experiment with different greens, such as kale or Swiss chard, to mix things up.

- Enjoy this smoothie as a refreshing breakfast option or as a mid-day snack for a healthy energy boost!

> *This Green Reset Smoothie is a delicious and nutritious way to reset your system while glowing with health.*

What does wellness mean to you today?

Day 1: Reclaim *Your Rhythm*

*Today, I choose to begin again—
with grace.*

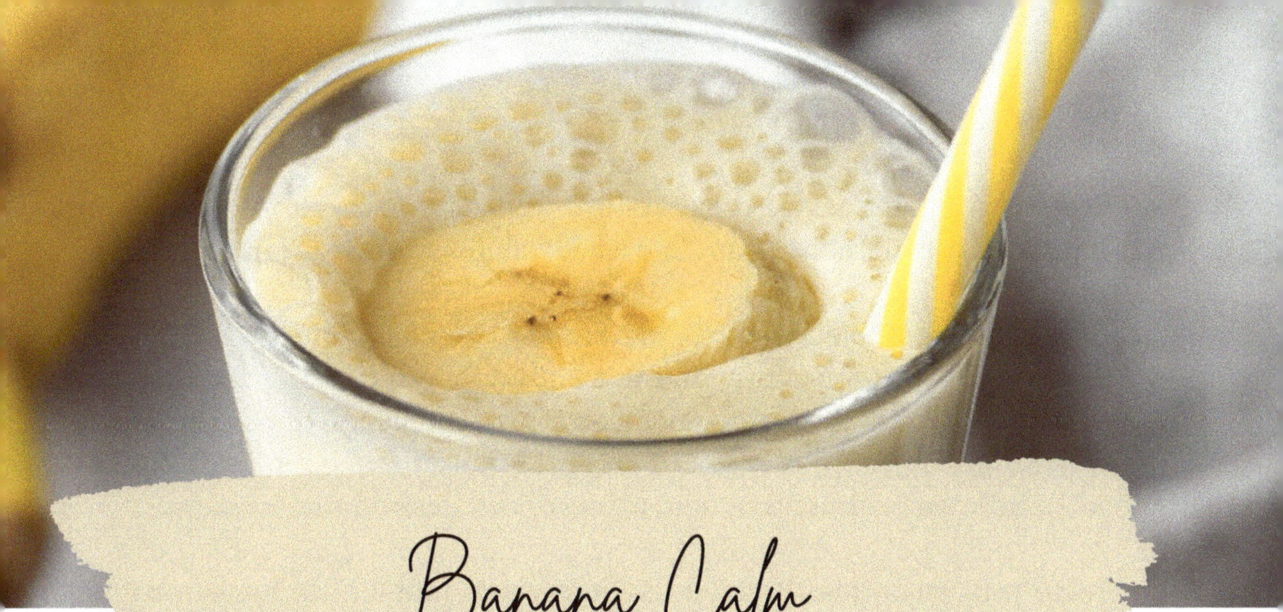

Banana Calm

Banana, almond milk, flaxseed, cinnamon, nut butter

The Banana Calm Smoothie is a creamy and comforting blend that's perfect for soothing bloating, stabilizing blood sugar, and supporting hormonal health. It's deliciously nutty and subtly spiced, making it a great addition to your afternoon repertoire.

INGREDIENTS:

- 1 ripe banana
- 1 cup unsweetened almond milk
- 1 tablespoon ground flaxseed
- 1/2 teaspoon ground cinnamon
- 1 tablespoon nut butter (almond, peanut, or cashew)
- Optional

OPTIONAL ADD-INS:

A splash of vanilla extract for added flavor or a pinch of sea salt to enhance the sweetness.

INSTRUCTIONS:

1. Peel the ripe banana and break it into chunks for more effortless blending. Gather all the ingredients and measure them out for convenience.

2. In a high-speed blender, add the banana chunks, almond milk, ground flaxseed, ground cinnamon, and nut butter. If you're using vanilla extract or sea salt, add those as well. Blend on high until the mixture is smooth and creamy, about 30-45 seconds. If you find the smoothie too thick, you can add a little more almond milk to achieve your desired consistency.

3. Taste your smoothie. If you'd like it sweeter, add a little honey or maple syrup and blend again until thoroughly mixed. If you want it colder, toss in the ice cubes and blend again until smooth. Pour the smoothie into a glass or to-go bottle. If you've made enough, you can store leftovers in the fridge for up to 24 hours, but it's best enjoyed fresh. Garnish with a slice of lemon or an apple wedge if desired.

TIPS:

- For extra creaminess, consider adding a few frozen banana cubes instead of fresh ones.

- Experiment with different types of nut butters or even sunflower seed butter for a nut-free option. This smoothie can be made ahead of time and stored in the refrigerator for a few hours, but it's best enjoyed fresh to retain its optimal flavor and texture.

- The Banana Calm Smoothie is a delicious and nutritious way to help soothe your body while providing key nutrients that stabilize energy levels and support your overall well-being.

> *Enjoy your calming blend!*

What does wellness mean to you today?

Day 2: Detox *the Distractions*

> *Choosing yourself is not selfish; it is necessary for your growth.*

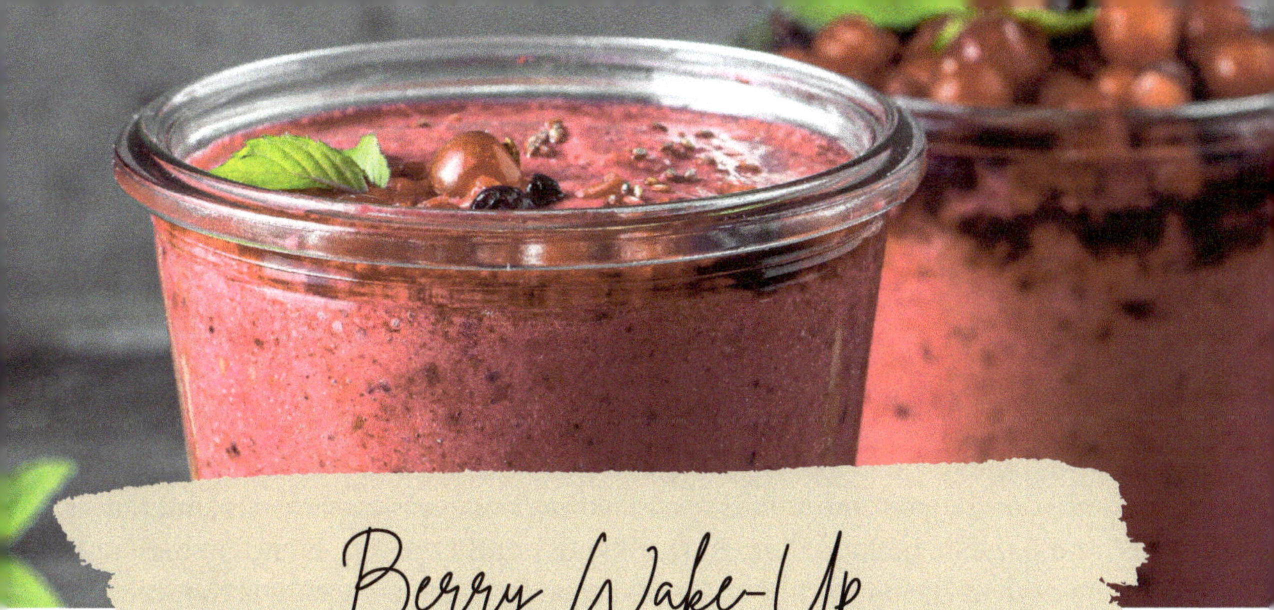

Berry Wake-Up

Blueberries, kale, chia seeds, lemon, coconut water

Kickstart your day with the Berry Wake-Up Smoothie! This vibrant and nutritious drink combines the sweetness of blueberries, the nutrient-dense properties of kale, and the hydrating benefits of coconut water. It's perfect for boosting your energy and providing essential vitamins and minerals.

INGREDIENTS:

- 1 ripe banana
- 1 cup unsweetened almond milk
- 1 tablespoon ground flaxseed
- 1/2 teaspoon ground cinnamon
- 1 tablespoon nut butter (almond, peanut, or cashew)
- Optional

OPTIONAL ADD-INS:

- 1 tablespoon honey or maple syrup: For additional sweetness if desired.
- 1 tablespoon nut butter: For added creaminess and healthy fats.
- 1/2 banana: For a sweeter, creamier texture.
- Ice cubes: For a colder, frostier smoothie.

INSTRUCTIONS:

1. If using fresh kale, wash the leaves well under cold water to remove any dirt. Remove the tough stems and tear the leaves into smaller pieces. If you're using fresh blueberries, rinse them under cold water. If you have frozen blueberries, there's no need to thaw them. Squeeze the juice from the lemon into a small bowl and set aside.

2. In a high-speed blender, add the blueberries, kale leaves, chia seeds, lemon juice, and coconut water. If you're adding honey or maple syrup, nut butter, or a banana, include them in the blender at this point. Blend on high until smooth and creamy, about 30-60 seconds. If the smoothie is too thick for your liking, you can add more coconut water or a splash of regular water to adjust the consistency.

3. After blending, taste your smoothie. If you prefer a sweeter taste, consider adding more honey or maple syrup and blending again. For a slightly tarter flavor, add an extra squeeze of lemon juice. Pour the smoothie into a glass or a to-go container. For an added touch, consider garnishing with a few whole blueberries or a sprinkle of chia seeds on top. For an extra-chilled drink, blend in 1 or 2 ice cubes before serving.

TIPS:

- For a creamier smoothie, try adding half an avocado, which also enhances the nutritional profile.

- Feel free to substitute kale for spinach if you prefer a milder flavor.

- This smoothie can be made ahead of time and stored in the refrigerator for a few hours, but it tastes best when freshly prepared.

> *Enjoy your Berry Wake-Up Smoothie as a delicious and energizing way to start your day!*

Day 2: Detox the Distractions

I am allowed to take up space.

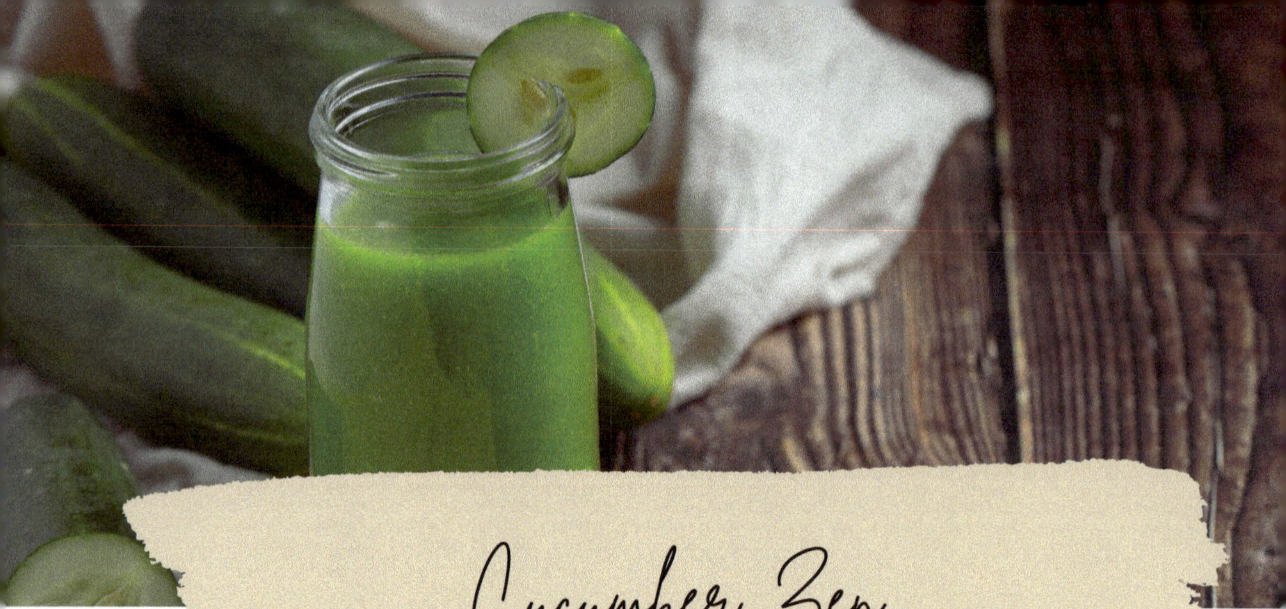

Cucumber Zen

Cucumber, mint, pear, lime, aloe juice

The Cucumber Zen Smoothie is a refreshing and revitalizing drink that combines hydrating cucumber, invigorating mint, sweet pear, zesty lime, and soothing aloe juice. This smoothie is not only delicious but also packed with nutrients that promote hydration and digestion, making it an ideal choice for a hot day or a post-workout refreshment.

INGREDIENTS:

- 1 medium cucumber
- 1 ripe pear
- 1/2 cup fresh mint leaves
- Juice of 1 lime
- 1/2 cup aloe vera juice

OPTIONAL ADD-INS:

- 1 tablespoon honey or agave syrup: For added sweetness, if desired.
- ½ cup ice cubes for a chilled smoothie.
- A few slices of fresh ginger for an extra zing and digestive benefits.

INSTRUCTIONS:

1. Wash the cucumber thoroughly and cut it into chunks. You can peel it if you prefer a milder flavor, but keeping the skin on adds extra nutrients. Wash the fresh mint leaves and gently pat them dry. Core and chop the pear into chunks, leaving the skin on for added fiber. Squeeze the juice from the lime using a citrus juicer and set it aside.

2. In a high-speed blender, combine the cucumber chunks, pear pieces, fresh mint leaves, lime juice, and aloe vera juice. If you're using honey or agave syrup for extra sweetness, add it now. For a colder smoothie, add the ice cubes (if using). Blend on high until smooth and creamy, about 30-45 seconds.

3. Taste your smoothie and adjust as needed. If you'd like it to be sweeter, add more honey or agave syrup and blend again. For a stronger mint flavor, consider adding a few more mint leaves and mixing again. Pour the smoothie into glasses or a to-go container. Garnish with a sprig of mint or a slice of cucumber on the rim of the glass if desired.

TIPS:

- For added creaminess, consider blending in a spoonful of yogurt or a ripe avocado.

- Experiment with other herbs, such as basil or cilantro, for unique flavors.

- This smoothie is best enjoyed fresh but can be stored in the refrigerator for a short time; give it a good shake before drinking.

- This Cucumber Zen Smoothie is the perfect way to start your day or refresh yourself during a hot afternoon.

> *Enjoy the invigorating flavors and health benefits it brings!*

How can I show up for myself today?

Day 3: Breathe & Reset

In the chaos of life, find your calm and shine your light.

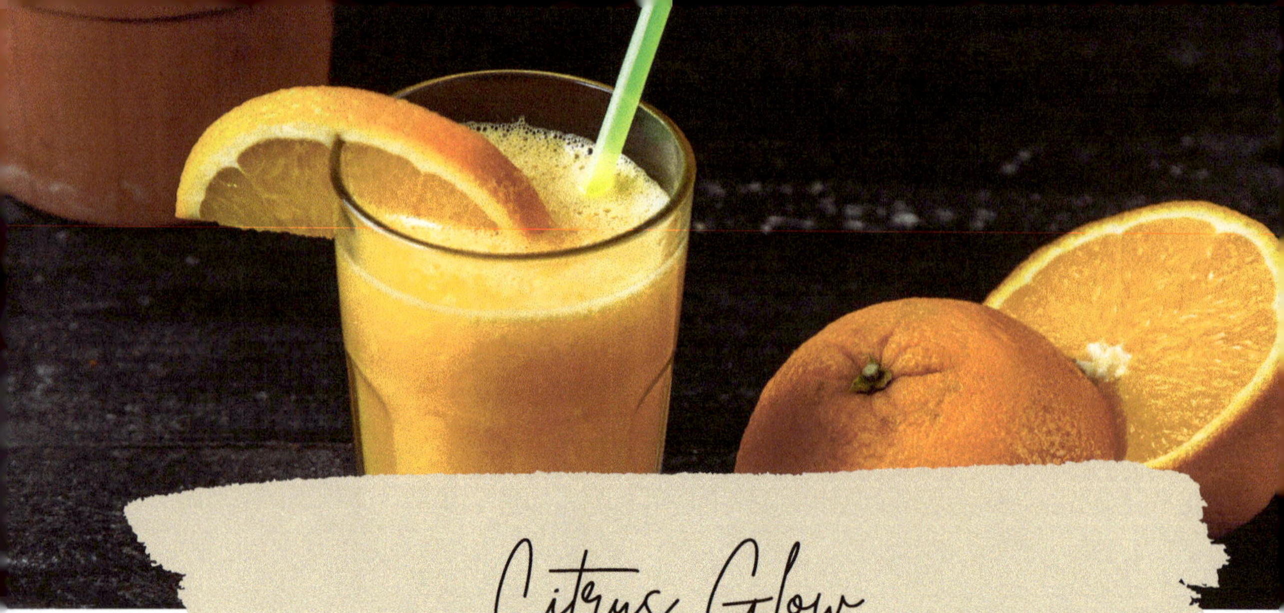

Citrus Glow

Orange, pineapple, turmeric, ginger, filtered water

The Citrus Glow Smoothie is a vibrant and refreshing drink packed with vitamins, antioxidants, and anti-inflammatory properties. This smoothie combines the tangy sweetness of oranges and pineapples with the warming spices of turmeric and ginger, making it perfect for a morning boost or a mid-afternoon refresher.

INGREDIENTS:

- 1 large orange
- 1 cup fresh pineapple chunks
- 1/2 teaspoon ground turmeric
- ½ inch piece of fresh ginger
- 1 cup filtered water

OPTIONAL ADD-INS:

- 1 tablespoon honey or maple syrup: For additional sweetness if desired.
- 1/4 avocado: For creaminess and healthy fats.
- A few ice cubes: To chill your smoothie.
- 1 tablespoon chia seeds or flaxseed: For added fiber and omega-3 fatty acids.

INSTRUCTIONS:

1. Peel the orange and separate it into segments, removing any seeds as you go. If using fresh pineapple, cut it into chunks. If using canned or frozen, make sure it's properly drained and thawed if frozen. Peel the ginger piece and slice it into smaller chunks for more effortless blending. Gather all your ingredients for easy access while blending.

2. In a high-speed blender, add the orange segments, pineapple chunks, ground turmeric, fresh ginger slices, and filtered water. If you're using optional add-ins like honey for sweetness, avocado for creaminess, or chia or flax seeds, add them at this stage as well. Blend on high until smooth and creamy, about 30-60 seconds. If the smoothie is too thick, feel free to add a little more water to reach your desired consistency.

3. Taste your smoothie. If you want it sweeter, add more honey or maple syrup and blend again. If you'd like a spicier kick, you can add a touch more ginger or a small pinch of black pepper to enhance the absorption of turmeric. Pour the smoothie into a tall glass or a to-go container. If desired, garnish with a slice of orange or sprinkle of turmeric on top.

TIPS:

- For added flavor complexity, consider adding a splash of coconut water for natural sweetness and electrolytes.

- For an extra boost of nutrients, you can toss in a handful of spinach or kale without significantly altering the flavor.

- This smoothie can be stored in the refrigerator for a few hours, but it's best consumed fresh to preserve its nutrients and flavor.

> *Enjoy the vibrant and health-boosting properties of your Citrus Glow Smoothie! It's a delicious way to support your immune system and fuel your day.*

Day 3: Breathe & Reset

Letting go is how I make room for more.

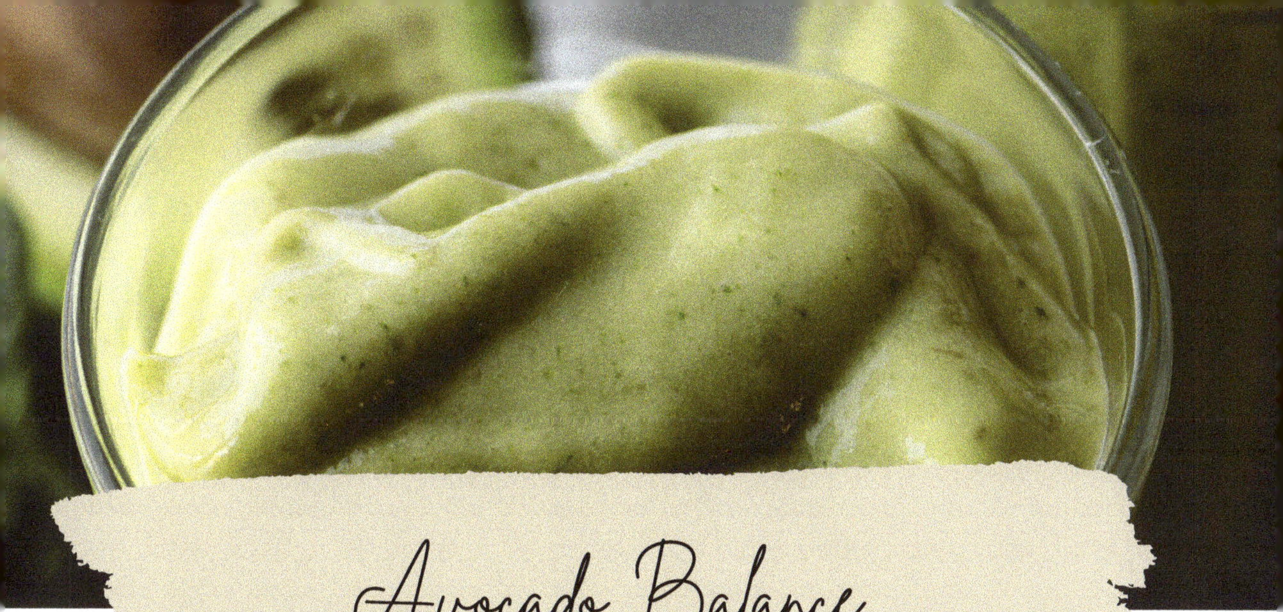

Avocado Balance

Avocado, banana, unsweetened oat milk, cinnamon

The Avocado Balance Smoothie is a creamy, nourishing blend that combines the rich texture of avocado with the natural sweetness of banana. This smoothie is perfect for promoting hormonal balance and supporting satiety due to its healthy fat content. The addition of unsweetened oat milk and a hint of cinnamon enhances the flavor while keeping it wholesome and satisfying.

INGREDIENTS:

- 1 ripe avocado
- 1 medium ripe banana
- 1 cup unsweetened oat milk
- 1/2 teaspoon ground cinnamon

OPTIONAL ADD-INS:

- 1 tablespoon honey or maple syrup: For extra sweetness, if desired.
- 1 tablespoon chia seeds or flaxseed: For added fiber and omega-3 fatty acids.
- Ice cubes: For a colder, refreshing smoothie.

INSTRUCTIONS:

1. Cut the avocado in half, remove the pit, and scoop the flesh into the blender. Peel the banana and break it into chunks for more effortless blending. Gather your oat milk, cinnamon, and any optional ingredients you plan to use.

2. In a high-speed blender, add the avocado flesh, banana chunks, unsweetened oat milk, and cinnamon. If you're using optional ingredients like honey or maple syrup, chia seeds, or flaxseed, add them to the blender. For added chill, you can include a few ice cubes.

3. Blend on high speed until all ingredients are smooth and creamy. This should take about 30-60 seconds. If the mixture is too thick for your liking, add more oat milk until you reach your preferred consistency.

TIPS:

- For a protein boost, consider adding a scoop of your favorite protein powder.

- This smoothie can be a great breakfast option or a post-workout snack.

- If you're using frozen bananas, there's no need for ice cubes, as the frozen fruit will keep your smoothie chilled.

> *Enjoy your creamy and satisfying Avocado Balance Smoothie, perfect for promoting hormonal health and keeping you feeling full throughout the day!*

What can I let go of today?

Day 4: Calm the Gut

Celebrate progress, not perfection, every small step counts.

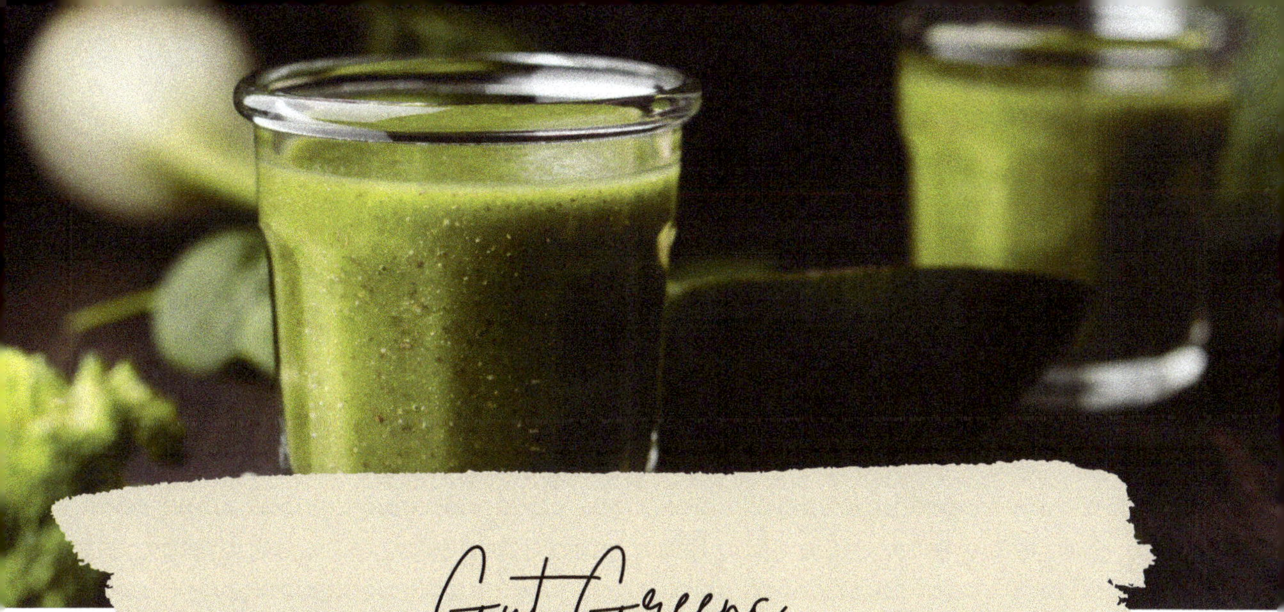

Gut Greens

Celery, green apple, romaine, lemon, ginger

The Gut Greens Smoothie is a refreshing and nutrient-dense drink designed to support digestive health and promote an alkaline internal environment. This vibrant green smoothie is packed with gut-friendly ingredients like celery, green apple, and ginger, making it an excellent choice for a morning boost or a healthy snack.

INGREDIENTS:

- 2 stalks of celery
- 1 green apple
- 2 cups romaine lettuce
- Juice of 1 lemon
- 1-inch piece of fresh ginger

OPTIONAL ADD-INS:

- 1 tablespoon chia seeds or flaxseeds: For added fiber and omega-3 fatty acids.
- 1/2 cucumber: For additional hydration and a refreshing flavor.
- 1 teaspoon honey or maple syrup: For those who prefer a sweeter taste.
- Ice cubes: For a colder, refreshing smoothie.

INSTRUCTIONS:

1. Wash the celery stalks thoroughly, then chop them into smaller pieces for more effortless blending. Rinse the green apple, core it, and chop it into quarters (you can leave the skin on for added fiber). Wash the romaine lettuce leaves and tear them into smaller pieces. Peel the ginger and slice it into smaller chunks for more effortless blending. Cut the lemon in half and squeeze out the juice using a citrus juicer or a fork, discarding the seeds.

2. In a high-speed blender, combine the chopped celery, green apple pieces, romaine lettuce, ginger, and lemon juice. Add about 1 cup of filtered water (adjust the amount as needed to achieve your desired consistency). Blend on high speed until smooth and creamy, about 30 to 60 seconds. If the mixture is too thick, add more water until you reach your preferred consistency.

TIPS:

- Experiment with adding other leafy greens, like spinach or kale, for added nutrients without significantly altering the flavor.
- If you prefer a colder smoothie, use frozen fruit or add ice cubes before blending.
- This smoothie can be made ahead of time and stored in the refrigerator for a few hours, but it's best enjoyed fresh for optimal flavor and nutrients.

> *Enjoy your refreshing Gut Greens Smoothie as a delicious way to support your digestive health and nourish*

Day 4: Calm the Gut

I honor my body by listening to its whispers.

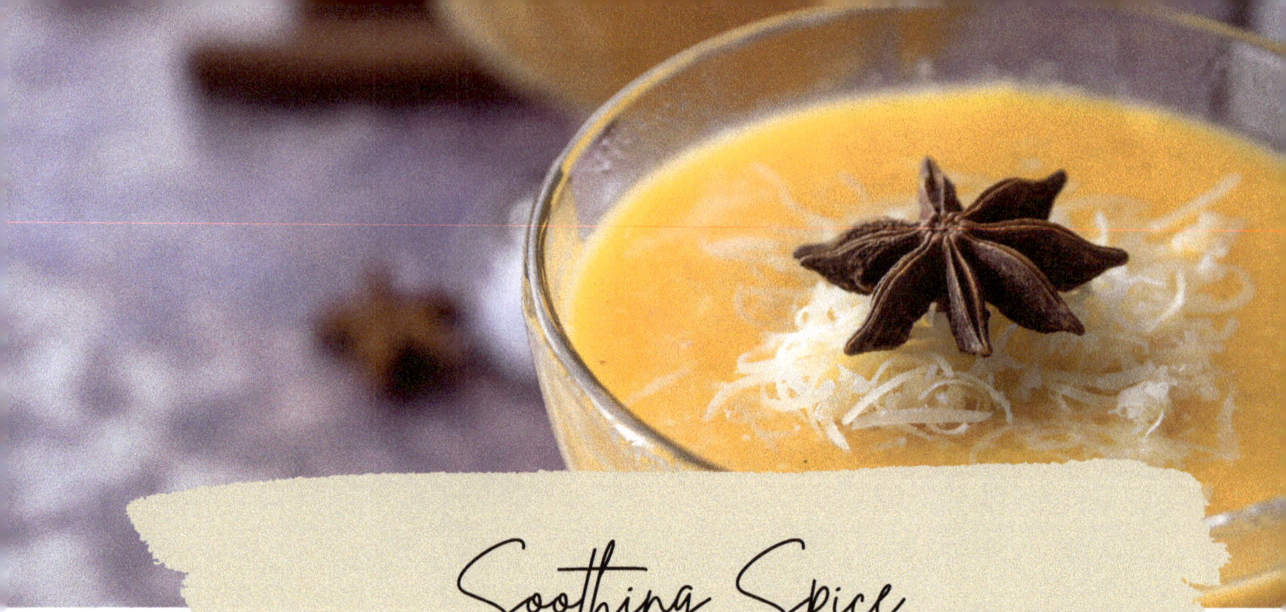

Soothing Spice

Pumpkin purée, almond milk, nutmeg, cinnamon, chia seeds

The Soothing Spice Smoothie is a cozy, warm blend that's perfect for relaxing your body and mind before bedtime. Combining creamy pumpkin purée with soothing spices like nutmeg and cinnamon, this smoothie is rich in fiber and will help put you in a restful mood.

The addition of almond milk and chia seeds creates a creamy texture while providing essential nutrients to help promote a peaceful night's sleep.

INGREDIENTS:

- 1/2 cup pumpkin purée
- 1 cup unsweetened almond milk
- 1/2 teaspoon ground nutmeg
- 1/2 teaspoon ground cinnamon
- 2 tablespoons chia seeds

OPTIONAL ADD-INS:

- 1 tablespoon honey or maple syrup: For additional sweetness if desired.
- A pinch of sea salt: To enhance the flavors.
- 1/4 teaspoon vanilla extract: For added depth of flavor.
- Ice cubes: If you prefer your smoothie chilled

INSTRUCTIONS:

1. Measure out the pumpkin purée. If using canned pumpkin, ensure it is 100% pure pumpkin and not pumpkin pie filling, which contains added sugars and spices. Measure out the almond milk and set it aside. Gather and measure the nutmeg, cinnamon, chia seeds, and any optional add-ins.

2. In a high-speed blender, add the pumpkin purée, almond milk, ground nutmeg, ground cinnamon, and chia seeds. If you prefer a chilled version, you can also add a few ice cubes. Blend on high until the mixture is smooth and creamy, which should take about 30-60 seconds. The chia seeds will also begin to soften and slightly thicken the smoothie. Stop the blender scrape down the sides if necessary, and blend again if needed to reach your desired consistency.

TIPS:

- For a creamier texture, consider blending in a few tablespoons of Greek yogurt or a banana.

- This smoothie is perfect for winding down after a long day—enjoy it in a calm setting to maximize relaxation.

- If you're preparing the smoothie ahead of time, keep in mind that the chia seeds will absorb some liquid over time, thickening the mixture.

- You might need to add a little extra almond milk to thin it out before drinking.

> *Enjoy your soothing, cozy Soothing Spice Smoothie as an excellent way to promote relaxation and nourishment before bedtime!*

Where do I see beauty in myself at this moment?

Day 5: Flush the Fog

Wellness is a journey, not a destination-enjoy the ride.

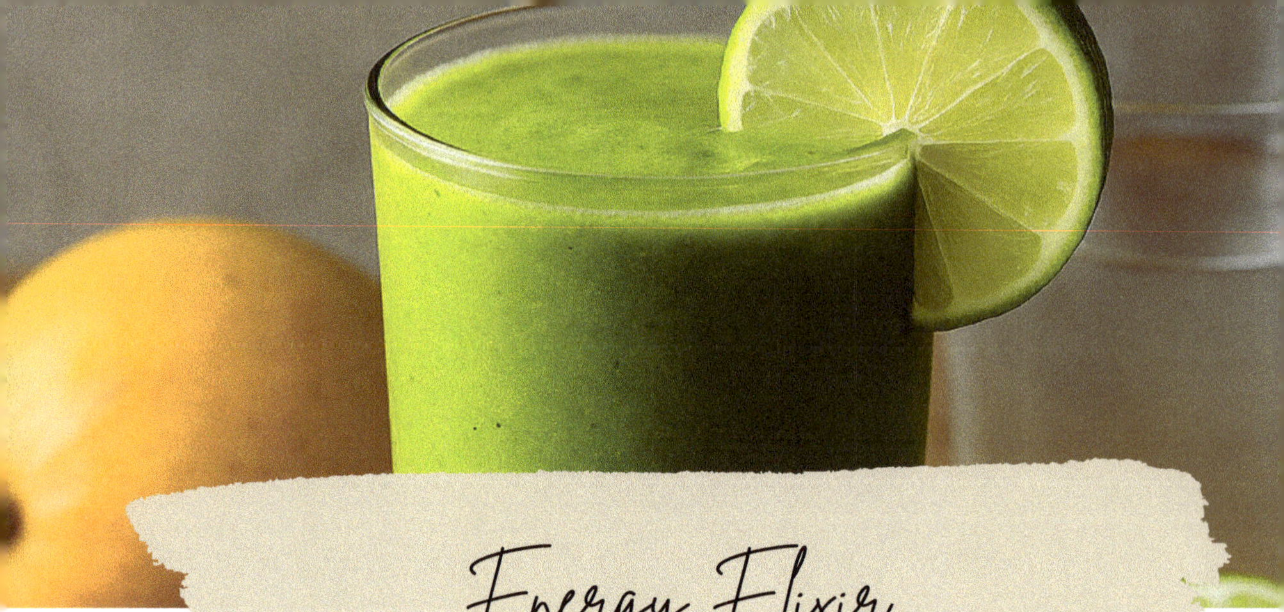

Energy Elixir

Mango, coconut water, spinach, lime

The Energy Elixir is a vibrant and refreshing smoothie designed to hydrate, energize, and support brain function. Combining the sweetness of mango with the hydration of coconut water, the nutritional benefits of spinach, and the zesty kick of lime, this smoothie is perfect for a morning boost or an afternoon pick-me-up.

INGREDIENTS:

- 1 ripe mango
- 1 cup coconut water
- 2 cups fresh spinach
- Juice of 1 lime

OPTIONAL ADD-INS:

- 1 tablespoon chia seeds or flaxseeds: For added fiber and omega-3 fatty acids, which support brain health.
- 1/2 banana: For extra creaminess and natural sweetness if preferred.
- A handful of ice cubes: For a colder, thicker smoothie.
- 1 tablespoon honey or agave syrup: For added sweetness.

INSTRUCTIONS:

1. If using a fresh mango, peel it, remove the pit, and cut it into chunks. If you're using frozen mango, no preparation is needed. Measure out your coconut water, spinach, and lime juice (squeezed from the lime). Gather any optional ingredients you plan to use.

2. In a high-speed blender, add the mango chunks, coconut water, fresh spinach, and lime juice. If you're including optional ingredients like chia seeds, flaxseeds, or honey, add them. For a colder and thicker smoothie, add a handful of ice cubes. Blend on high until the mixture is completely smooth and creamy. This should take about 30-60 seconds. Stop and scrape down the sides if necessary to ensure all ingredients are well-blended.

TIPS:

- This smoothie is perfect for post-workout recovery due to its high hydration and nutrient content.

- Feel free to experiment with other greens, like kale or Swiss chard, to vary the nutrient profile.

- You can prepare ingredients ahead of time and freeze the mango for a quick smoothie option.

> *Enjoy your refreshing and revitalizing Energy Elixir as a delicious way to fuel your day!*

Day 5:
Flush *the Fog*

*"This moment is mine.
I reclaim it with love."*

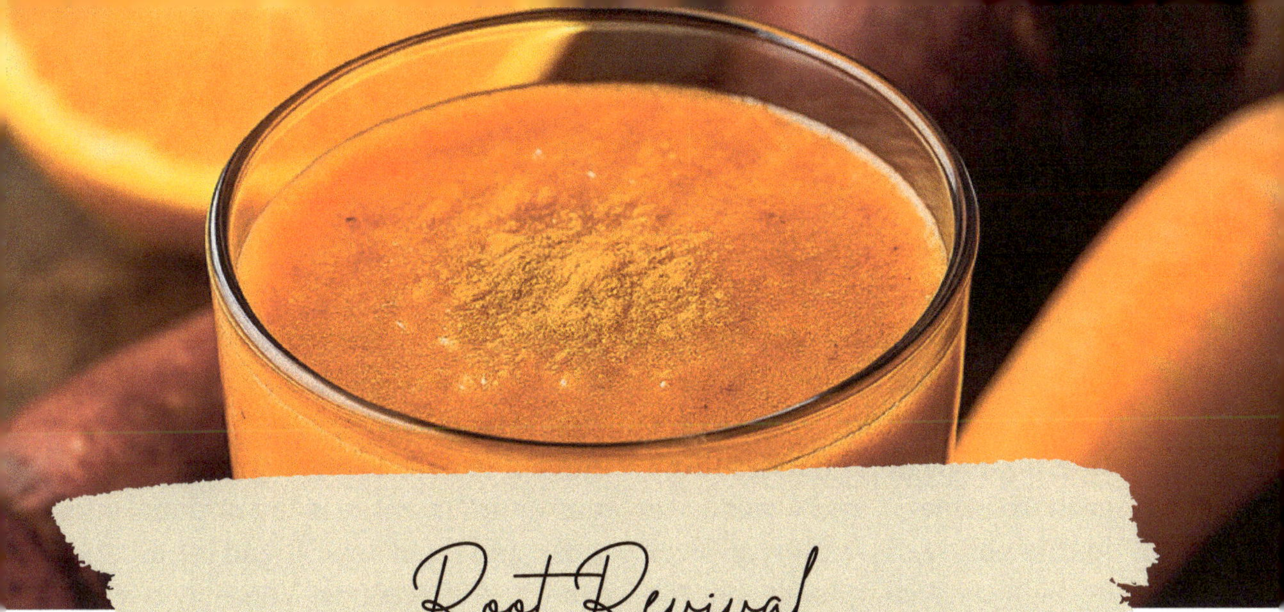

Root Revival

Carrot, beet, orange, turmeric

The Root Revival Smoothie is a vibrant and nutritious drink that combines the goodness of carrots, beets, and oranges, along with the anti-inflammatory benefits of turmeric. This smoothie is designed to improve circulation, detoxify the liver, and provide you with a natural energy boost. The earthy flavors of the roots, combined with the citrusy brightness, make this a delightful and healthful choice.

INGREDIENTS:

- 1 medium carrot
- 1 small beet
- 1 large orange
- 1/2 teaspoon ground turmeric
- 1 cup water or coconut water

OPTIONAL ADD-INS:

- 1 tablespoon chia seeds or flaxseeds: For added fiber and omega-3 fatty acids.
- 1 teaspoon honey or maple syrup: For those who prefer a sweeter taste.
- A pinch of black pepper: To enhance the absorption of turmeric's active compound, curcumin.
- A handful of ice cubes: For a chilled smoothie if desired.

INSTRUCTIONS:

1. Peel and chop the carrot into smaller pieces for more effortless blending. If using a fresh beet, peel it, then chop it into small cubes. If you're using pre-cooked or canned beets, rinse and drain them well. Peel the orange and separate it into segments, ensuring you remove any seeds. Gather your turmeric, water, coconut water, and any optional ingredients.

2. In a high-speed blender, add the chopped carrot, beet, orange segments, ground turmeric, and water or coconut water. If you're using optional add-ins like chia seeds, honey, or black pepper, add them now. Blend the mixture on high until completely smooth, about 30-60 seconds. You may need to stop and scrape down the sides to ensure everything is well-blended. If the smoothie is too thick, you can add more water or coconut water to achieve your desired consistency.

TIPS:

- To enhance the detoxification benefits, consider adding a handful of spinach or kale for added nutrients.

- If you enjoy a bit of sweetness without added sugars, a frozen banana can provide a creamy texture and natural sweetness.

- This smoothie is an excellent way to start your day, recover after a workout, or enjoy it as a revitalizing afternoon snack.

> *Enjoy the invigorating and health-boosting benefits of your Root Revival Smoothie!*

What feels better in my body this week?

Day 6:
Choose *You Again*

Your purpose is not what you do but who you are becoming.

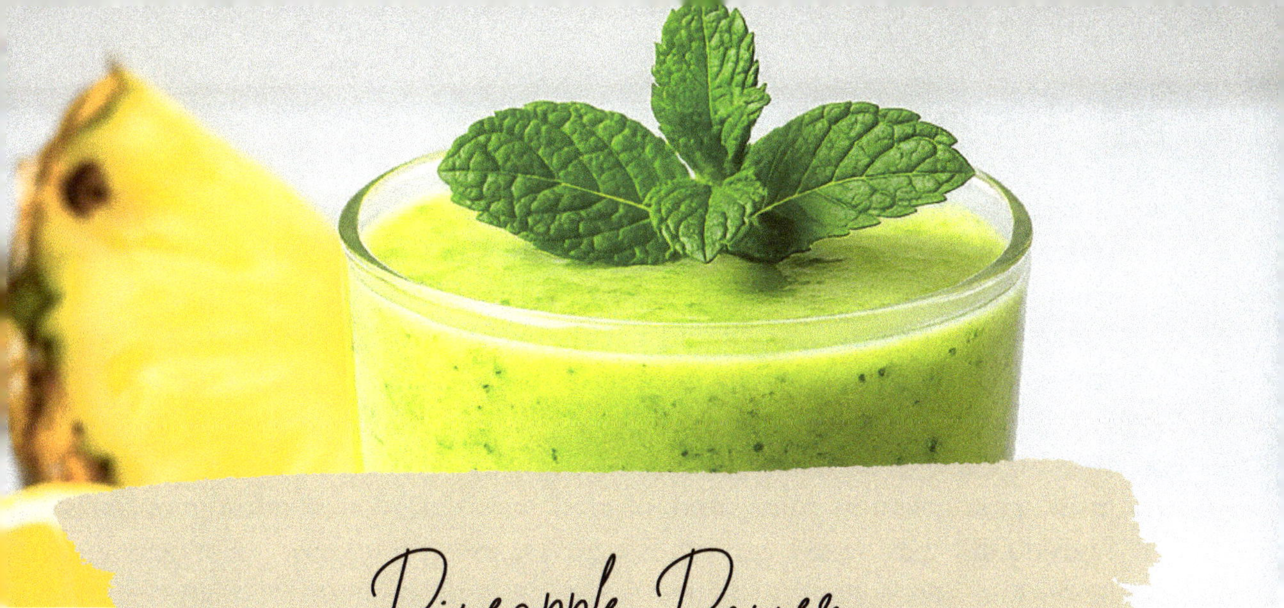

Pineapple Power

Pineapple, cucumber, mint, lemon, filtered water

The Pineapple Power Smoothie is a refreshing and revitalizing drink designed to help you feel less bloated while uplifting your mood. The combination of sweet pineapple, hydrating cucumber, cool mint, and zesty lemon creates a delicious tropical smoothie that not only tastes great but also supports hydration and digestion.

INGREDIENTS:

- 1 cup fresh pineapple chunks
- 1/2 medium cucumber
- 1/4 cup fresh mint leaves
- Juice of 1 lemon
- 1 cup filtered water

OPTIONAL ADD-INS:

- 1 tablespoon honey or maple syrup: For a sweeter taste.
- 1 tablespoon chia seeds or flaxseeds: For added fiber and omega-3 fatty acids.
- Ice cubes: For a colder, refreshing smoothie.

INSTRUCTIONS:

1. If using fresh pineapple, peel, core, and chop it into chunks. If using frozen pineapple, there's no need to thaw. Wash the cucumber thoroughly and chop it into smaller pieces. You can peel it if you prefer a milder flavor. Rinse the fresh mint leaves and pat them dry. Cut the lemon in half and squeeze out the juice using a juicer or a fork, discarding any seeds.

2. In a high-speed blender, combine the pineapple chunks, cucumber, fresh mint leaves, lemon juice, and filtered water. If you're adding optional ingredients like honey or chia seeds, include them now. For a colder smoothie, add a handful of ice cubes. Blend on high for about 30-60 seconds or until the mixture is smooth and creamy. If necessary, stop and scrape down the sides to ensure everything is well blended. If the smoothie appears too thick, you can add more filtered water to reach your desired consistency.

TIPS:

- This smoothie is perfect for hot days or after a workout to replenish hydration.

- Feel free to experiment with other herbs, such as basil, for a unique twist on flavor.

- Enjoy this smoothie as a refreshing snack or healthy breakfast option to start your day on a positive note!

> *Enjoy your revitalizing and uplifting Pineapple Power Smoothie!*

Day 6:
Choose *You Again*

Small shifts birth powerful change.

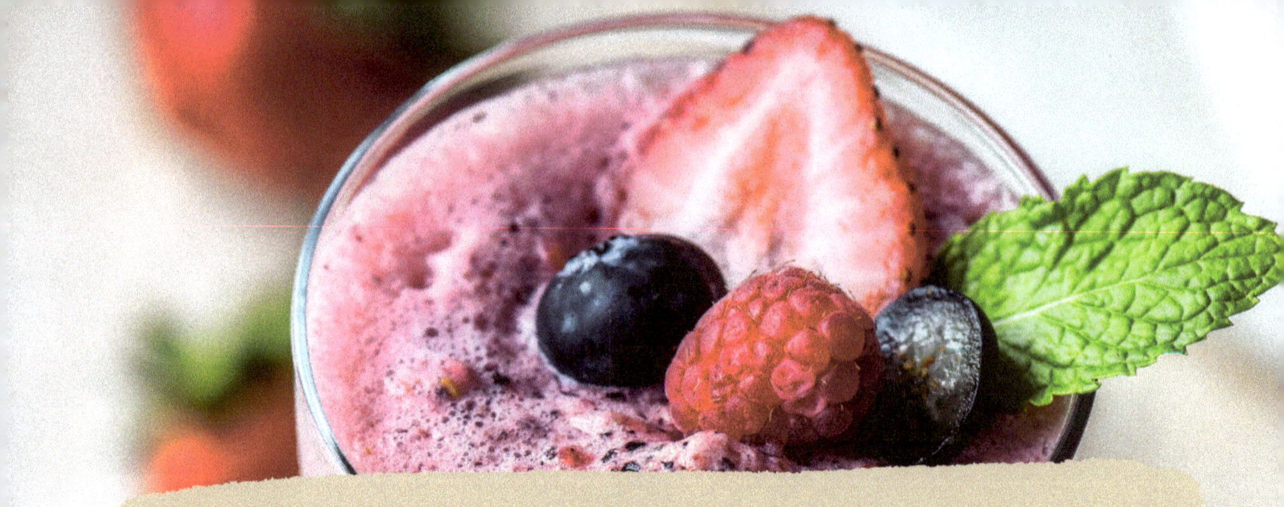

Hormone Helper

Berries, ground flax, kale, almond milk

The Hormone Helper Smoothie is a nourishing blend specifically designed to support hormone regulation and promote healthy skin. Packed with antioxidant-rich berries, fiber from ground flaxseed, and nutrient-dense kale, this smoothie is both delicious and beneficial for overall wellness. The creamy almond milk ties everything together for a satisfying and refreshing drink.

INGREDIENTS:

- 1 cup mixed berries (fresh or frozen)
- 2 tablespoons ground flaxseed
- 1 cup fresh kale leaves
- 1 cup unsweetened almond milk

OPTIONAL ADD-INS:

- 1 tablespoon honey or maple syrup: For added sweetness, if desired.
- 1 banana: For extra creaminess and natural sweetness.
- 1/2 tablespoon chia seeds: For additional fiber and omega-3s.
- A pinch of cinnamon: For flavor and added health benefits.

INSTRUCTIONS:

1. Wash the mixed berries thoroughly (if using fresh). If you're using frozen berries, you can use them directly from the freezer. Rinse the kale leaves and remove the stems. Tear the leaves into smaller pieces for more effortless blending. Measure out the ground flaxseed and almond milk. Combine Ingredients in

2. In a high-speed blender, add the mixed berries, ground flaxseed, kale leaves, and almond milk. If you're using optional add-ins like honey, banana, chia seeds, or cinnamon, add them as desired. Blend on high until the mixture is smooth and creamy, about 30-60 seconds. You may need to stop and scrape down the sides to ensure all ingredients are well incorporated. If the smoothie is too thick, add a bit more almond milk to adjust the consistency to your liking.

TIPS:

- This smoothie makes an excellent breakfast option or a refreshing afternoon snack.

- You can swap out kale for spinach if you prefer a milder flavor.

- For added protein, consider incorporating a scoop of your favorite protein powder.

> *Enjoy this delicious and nutrient-rich Hormone Helper Smoothie as part of your wellness routine!*

What change in myself am I learning to welcome?

Day 7: Soft *Reset*

Nourish your mind, body, and spirit, and watch your life transform.

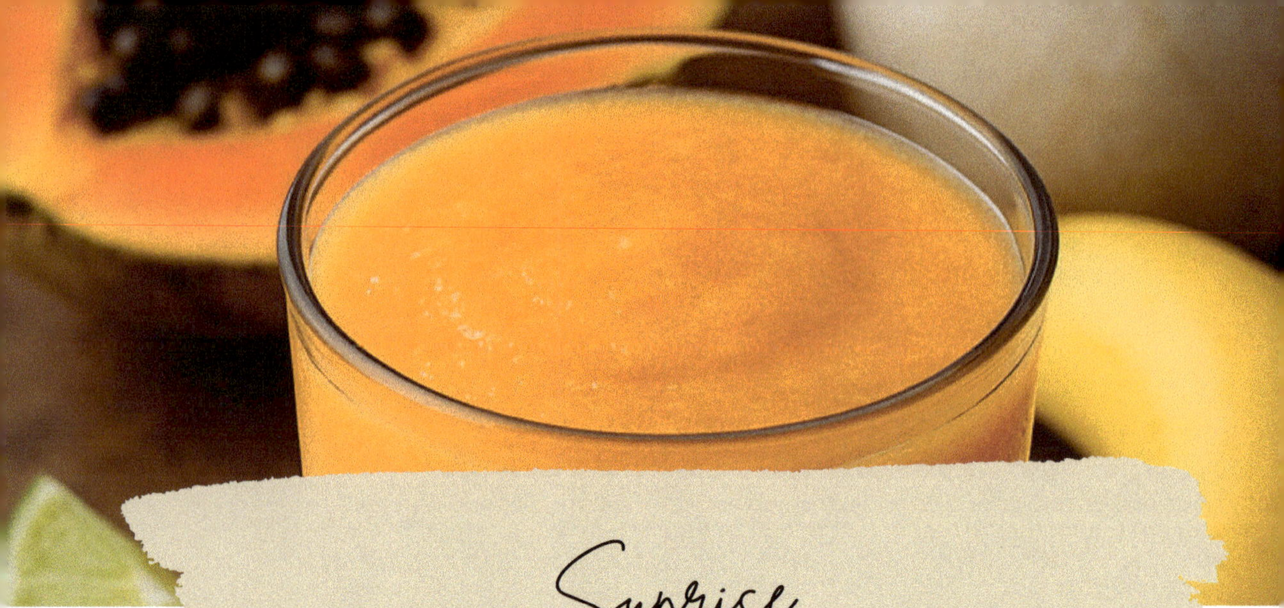

Sunrise

Papaya, banana, lime, coconut water

The Sunrise Smoothie is a vibrant, tropical blend that combines the sweetness of papaya and banana with the zesty brightness of lime, all balanced by the hydrating power of coconut water. This refreshing smoothie is designed to soothe digestion and promote a glowing complexion, making it a perfect choice for starting your day on a healthy note.

INGREDIENTS:

- 1 cup ripe papaya, peeled and diced
- 1 medium
- Juice of 1 lime
- 1 cup coconut water

INSTRUCTIONS:

1. If using fresh papaya, peel it, remove the seeds, and cut it into cubes. Peel the banana and break it into smaller pieces for more effortless blending. Cut the lime in half and squeeze out the juice, discarding any seeds. Measure out the coconut water and prepare any optional add-ins as needed.

2. In a high-speed blender, add the diced papaya, banana pieces, lime juice, and coconut water. If using optional ingredients like chia seeds, flaxseeds, or leafy greens, toss them in now. For a chilled smoothie, add a handful of ice cubes. Blend on high until the mixture is smooth and creamy, which should take about 30-60 seconds. Stop and scrape down the sides if necessary to ensure everything is well-blended.

3. If the smoothie is thicker than desired, you can add a small amount of coconut water or a splash of water to achieve your preferred consistency.

TIPS:

- This smoothie is a perfect way to start your day or as a refreshing afternoon snack.

- You can freeze papaya or banana slices ahead of time for a thicker and colder smoothie.

- Experiment by adding other tropical fruits, such as mango or pineapple, for a unique flavor profile.

> *Enjoy the refreshing and nourishing effects of your Sunrise Smoothie as you boost your digestion and achieve that radiant glow!*

Day 7: Soft *Reset*

This reset is sacred. So am I.

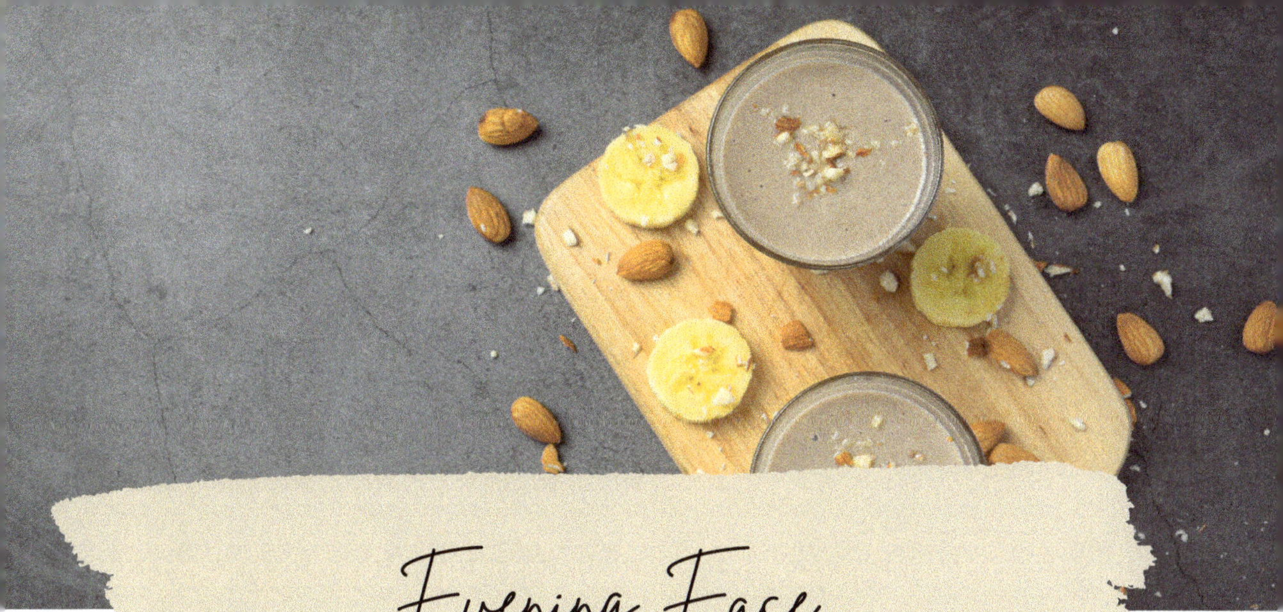

Evening Ease

Warm almond milk, dates, cinnamon, vanilla extract

The Evening Ease Smoothie is a warm and comforting blend perfect for winding down at the end of the day. This soothing drink features creamy almond milk, naturally sweet dates, fragrant cinnamon, and aromatic vanilla extract. It's designed to stabilize blood sugar levels before bed and promote relaxation, making it a delightful choice for a nighttime treat.

INGREDIENTS:

- 1 cup warm almond milk
- 2-3 Medjool dates
- 1/2 teaspoon ground cinnamon
- 1/2 teaspoon vanilla extract

INSTRUCTIONS:

1. Prepare the Almond Milk: In a small saucepan, warm the almond milk over low heat until it's warmed through but not boiling. Alternatively, heat it in the microwave for about 30-60 seconds.

2. Prepare the Dates: If your dates are not soft, consider soaking them in warm water for about 10 minutes to further soften them, which will help them blend more easily.

3. Combine Ingredients: In a high-speed blender, combine the warm almond milk, softened dates, ground cinnamon, and vanilla extract. If you're using any optional add-ins, toss them in as well.

4. Blend: Blend on high until the mixture is smooth and creamy. This should take about 30-45 seconds. Ensure that there are no chunks of dates remaining in the mix.

TIPS:

- For a richer, creamier texture, consider adding a spoonful of nut butter.
- This smoothie can also double as a warm digestif after dinner.
- Adjust the sweetness according to your taste preferences, and feel free to experiment with different spices.

Enjoy your warm and comforting Evening Ease Smoothie, perfect for promoting relaxation and stabilizing blood sugar before a restful night!

How can I honor rest today?

Reclaim & Cleanse Check-in

Return to yourself, release what no longer serves you, and realign with your body.

What parts of myself have I reclaimed this week—physically, emotionally, or spiritually? What am I beginning to hear or feel now that I've made space to listen?

Day 8:
Fuel *Your Fire*

Loving yourself is the greatest revolution you can create.

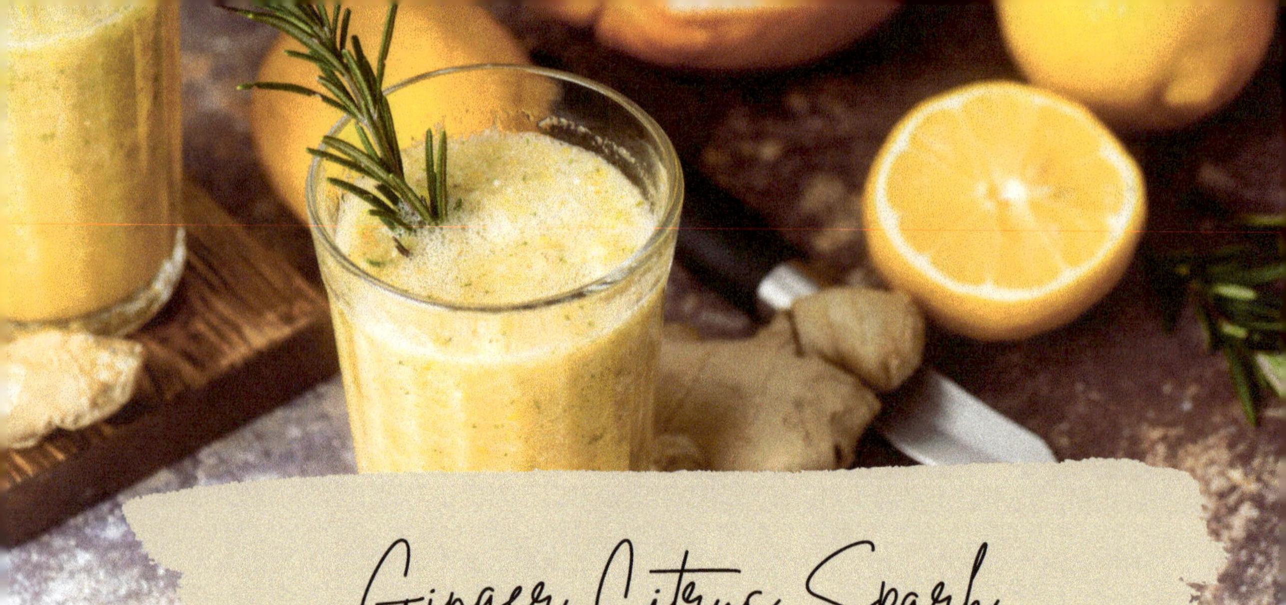

Ginger Citrus Spark

Orange, lemon, ginger, pineapple, coconut water

The Ginger Citrus Spark Smoothie is a vibrant and invigorating drink that combines the zesty flavors of orange and lemon with the warmth of ginger and the tropical sweetness of pineapple. This energizing smoothie is perfect for boosting your immune system and replenishing your hydration levels, making it a great choice to start your day or enjoy as an afternoon pick-me-up.

INGREDIENTS:

- 1 large orange, peeled and segmented
- 1/2 lemon, juiced
- 1-inch piece of fresh ginger, peeled and sliced
- 1 cup fresh pineapple chunks
- 1 cup coconut water

INSTRUCTIONS:

1. Peel the orange and break it into segments, removing any seeds as you go. Cut the lemon in half and squeeze out the juice, removing any seeds as you go. Peel the ginger and slice it thinly. If using fresh pineapple, peel, core, and cut it into chunks. If using frozen, you can add it directly.

2. In a high-speed blender, add the orange segments, lemon juice, ginger slices, pineapple chunks, and coconut water. If you're using optional ingredients like honey, banana, or leafy greens, add them to the blender. Blend on high until the mixture is smooth and creamy, about 30-60 seconds. Stop and scrape down the sides if necessary to ensure everything is well blended. If the smoothie is too thick, you can add more coconut water to reach your desired consistency. Taste your Ginger Citrus Spark Smoothie. If you want it sweeter, add more honcy or agave and blend again. For a stronger ginger flavor, consider adding a little fresher ginger and blending again. Pour the smoothie into a glass or a to-go container. You can garnish it with a slice of orange or a few pieces of pineapple if desired.

3. Enjoy immediately to get the most flavor and nutrition!

TIPS:

- This smoothie is perfect for warm weather or post-workout recovery.

- Feel free to personalize it by adding other fruits or greens based on your preference.

- Prepare the ingredients in advance and freeze the pineapple for a convenient smoothie when you need a quick energy boost!

Enjoy your refreshing and health-boosting Ginger Citrus Spark Smoothie!

“

Day 8:
Fuel *Your Fire*

My energy is precious—
I protect it with purpose.

”

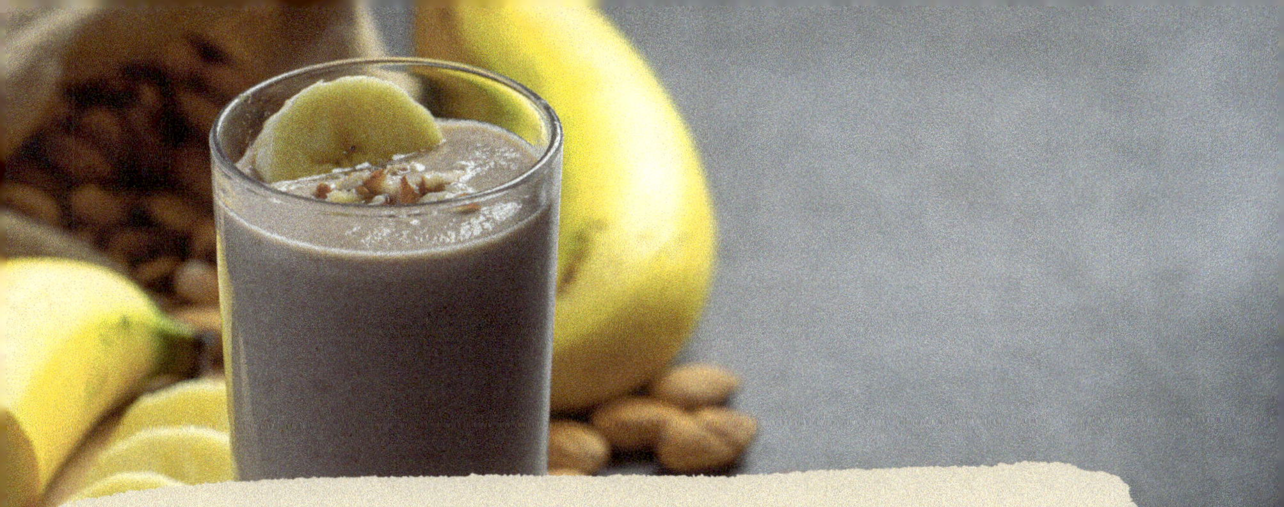

Almond Energy

Almond butter, banana, oat milk, dates, cinnamon

Almond Energy is a delicious and satisfying blend that's packed with protein and natural energy. The combination of almond butter, banana, oat milk, dates, and cinnamon creates a creamy, sweet, and smooth treat perfect for a post-workout snack or a healthy evening treat. The ingredients work synergistically to provide a great source of energy while keeping you fueled and satisfied.

INGREDIENTS:

- 2 tablespoons almond butter
- 1 medium ripe banana
- 1 cup unsweetened oat milk
- 3-4 Medjool dates
- 1/2 teaspoon ground cinnamon

OPTIONAL ADD-INS:

- 1 tablespoon chia seeds or flaxseeds: For additional fiber and omega-3 fatty acids.
- A scoop of protein powder: To further boost the protein content.
- A handful of spinach or kale: For added nutrients without affecting the flavor.
- Ice cubes: For a chilled, refreshing smoothie.

INSTRUCTIONS:

1. Peel the banana and break it into chunks for more effortless blending. If using whole dates, remove the pits and chop them into smaller pieces if necessary. Gather your almond butter, oat milk, cinnamon, and any optional ingredients you plan to use. In a high-speed blender, add the almond butter, banana, oat milk, dates, and ground cinnamon. If you're using optional ingredients, add them to the blender now.

2. Blend on high speed until the mixture is completely smooth and creamy, which should take about 30-60 seconds. If needed, stop to scrape down the sides to ensure everything is thoroughly blended. If the smoothie is too thick for your liking, add a little more oat milk to adjust the consistency.

3. Taste your Almond Energy Smoothie. If you prefer a sweeter taste, you can add another date or a drizzle of honey or maple syrup and blend briefly again. For a stronger cinnamon flavor, add a pinch more and blend. Pour the smoothie into a glass or a to-go container. If desired, you can sprinkle a little extra cinnamon on top for garnish.

4. Enjoy immediately for the best flavor and texture!

TIPS:

- This smoothie is perfect as a post-workout recovery drink or as a satisfying evening snack.

- You can prepare the ingredients ahead of time and store them in the fridge for a quick smoothie when you need an energy boost.

- Freeze bananas or use frozen dates for a creamier texture and a chilled smoothie.

> *Enjoy your Almond Energy Smoothie as a rich and nourishing way to power up your evening!*

Where am I holding stress in my body?

Day 9: Rise *Gently*

Your journey is uniquely yours; embrace it with an open heart.

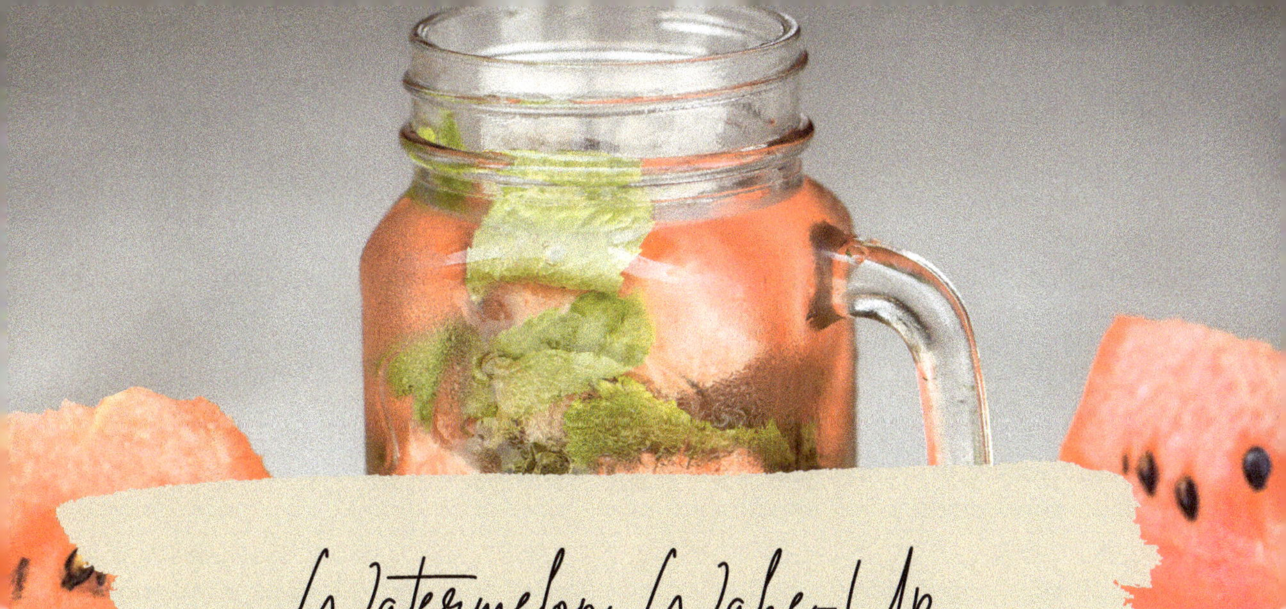

Watermelon Wake-Up

Watermelon, mint, lime, filtered water

The Watermelon Wake-Up Smoothie is a hydrating and refreshing drink that's perfect for a hot day or whenever you need a revitalizing boost. The combination of sweet watermelon, fresh mint, and zesty lime creates a deliciously light smoothie that will quench your thirst and energize you. Ideal for breakfast or as an afternoon pick-me-up, this smoothie is full of nutrients and flavor.

INGREDIENTS:

- 2 cups seedless watermelon, cubed
- 1/4 cup fresh mint leaves
- Juice of 1 lime
- 1 cup filtered water

OPTIONAL ADD-INS:

- 1 tablespoon chia seeds: For added fiber and omega-3 fatty acids.
- 1 tablespoon honey or agave syrup: For a sweeter smoothie.
- Ice cubes: For an extra chilled and refreshing smoothie.

INSTRUCTIONS:

1. If using fresh watermelon, cut it into cubes and remove any seeds. If using pre-cut watermelon, gather the pieces. Rinse the mint leaves thoroughly and pat them dry. Cut the lime in half and squeeze out the juice, discarding any seeds.

2. In a high-speed blender, add the watermelon cubes, fresh mint leaves, lime juice, and filtered water. If you're using any optional ingredients, such as chia seeds or honey, add them to the blender now. For a colder smoothie, feel free to add a few ice cubes.

3. Blend on high speed for 30-60 seconds or until the mixture is completely smooth and frothy. If needed, stop to scrape down the sides to ensure everything is well combined. If the smoothie is thicker than you prefer, add a little more filtered water to reach your desired consistency.

4. Taste your Watermelon Wake-Up Smoothie. If you prefer a sweeter taste, you can add a bit more honey or agave syrup and blend again. If you'd like a more pronounced lime flavor, feel free to squeeze in some extra lime juice.

5. Pour the smoothie into a glass or a to-go container. Garnish with a sprig of mint or a lime wedge for a decorative touch, if desired.

TIPS:

- This smoothie is perfect for hot summer days but can be enjoyed year-round.

- You can also experiment with other herbs, such as basil or a hint of ginger, for added flavor and health benefits.

- Make it a fun treat by freezing watermelon cubes beforehand for an extra frosty texture.

> *Enjoy your hydrating and refreshing Watermelon Wake-Up Smoothie!*

Day 9: Rise *Gently*

Rest is not weakness. It is wisdom.

Peach Recharge

Peach, spinach, avocado, almond milk

The Peach Recharge Smoothie is a delightful blend perfect for revitalizing your energy levels while providing hydration and healthy fats. The combination of juicy peaches, nutrient-dense spinach, creamy avocado, and smooth almond milk creates a refreshing, flavorful, and satisfying drink. This smoothie is excellent for breakfast, a midday snack, or a post-workout recovery.

INGREDIENTS:

- 1 ripe peach, pitted and chopped
- 1 cup fresh spinach
- 1/2 ripe avocado
- 1 cup unsweetened almond milk

OPTIONAL ADD-INS:

- 1 tablespoon chia seeds or flaxseeds: For added fiber and omega-3 fatty acids.
- 1 teaspoon honey or maple syrup: For extra sweetness if desired.
- 1/2 teaspoon vanilla extract: For added flavor.
- Ice cubes: For a cooler, refreshing smoothie.

INSTRUCTIONS:

1. Wash the peach, remove the pit, and chop it into small pieces. If using a frozen peach, make sure it is thawed slightly, or use it directly for a colder smoothie. Rinse the spinach leaves and pat them dry. Cut the avocado in half, remove the pit, and scoop out the flesh.

2. In a high-speed blender, add the chopped peach, fresh spinach, avocado, and almond milk. If you're using optional ingredients like chia seeds, honey, vanilla extract, or ice cubes, add them to the blender as well. Blend on high for 30-60 seconds or until the mixture is completely smooth and creamy. Stop to scrape down the sides if needed to ensure all ingredients are well combined. If the smoothie is too thick, you can add a little more almond milk to reach your desired consistency.

3. Taste your Peach Recharge Smoothie. If you want it sweeter, add a bit more honey or maple syrup and blend again. Adjust the amount of spinach if you prefer a stronger green flavor, but start with the original amount to maintain balance. Pour the smoothie into a glass or a to-go container. Garnish with a slice of peach or a few spinach leaves if desired.

TIPS:

- You can customize the smoothie by adding other fruits, such as berries or bananas, for an extra flavor and nutritional boost.

- This smoothie is perfect for a quick breakfast or a nutritious snack on the go.

- Freeze the peach beforehand for a colder, creamier smoothie.

> *Enjoy your refreshing Peach Recharge Smoothie, which balances hydration and healthy fats for sustained energy.*

What part of me needs gentleness (kindness) today?

Day 10: Feel the Flow

Happiness is a choice; choose to nourish your soul every day.

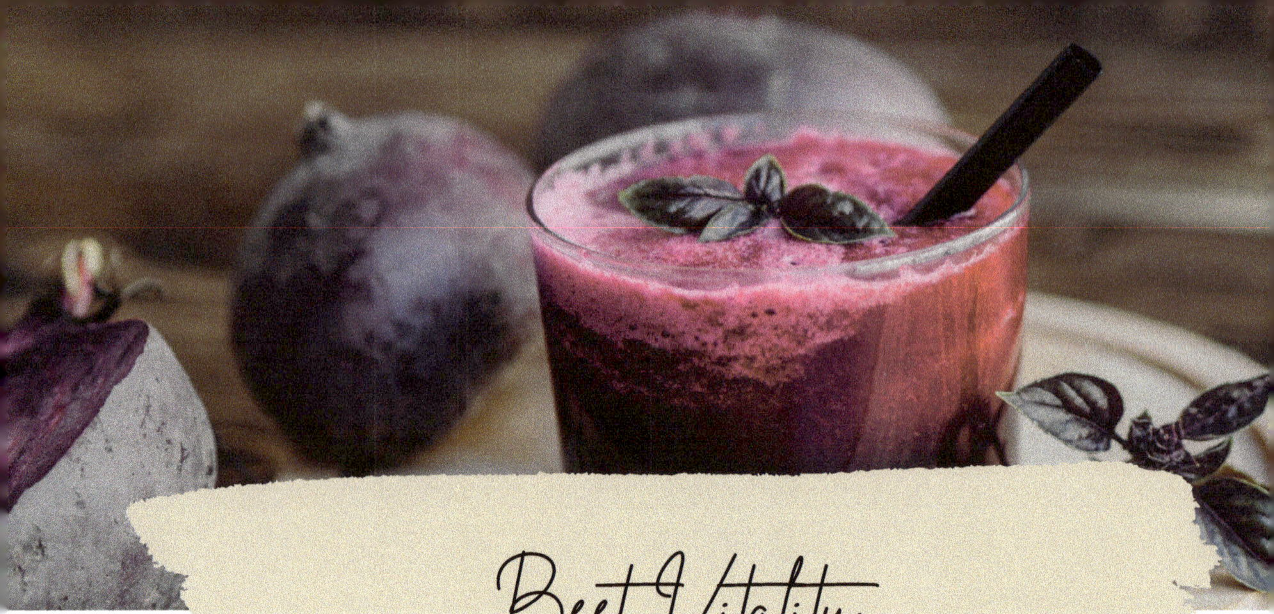

Beet Vitality

Beet, orange, ginger, lemon, filtered water

The Beet Vitality Smoothie is a vibrant and health-boosting drink that combines earthy beets, sweet oranges, zesty ginger, and tangy lemon. This smoothie is rich in antioxidants and nutrients designed to improve circulation and enhance stamina. It's perfect for anyone looking to energize their day or recover after a workout.

INGREDIENTS:

- 1 medium beet, peeled and chopped
- 1 large orange, peeled and segmented
- 1-inch piece of fresh ginger, peeled and sliced
- Juice of 1 lemon
- 1 cup filtered water

OPTIONAL ADD-INS:

- 1 tablespoon chia seeds or flaxseeds: For added fiber and omega-3 fatty acids.
- 1 tablespoon honey or maple syrup: If you prefer a sweeter taste.
- Ice cubes: For a chilled, refreshing smoothie.

INSTRUCTIONS:

1. Peel and chop the beet into small cubes (you can wear gloves to avoid staining your hands). Peel the orange and separate it into segments, ensuring that you remove all seeds. Peel the ginger and slice it into smaller pieces for more effortless blending. Cut the lemon in half and squeeze out the juice, discarding any seeds.

2. In a high-speed blender, add the chopped beet, orange segments, ginger slices, lemon juice, and filtered water. If you're using optional ingredients like chia seeds, honey, or ice cubes, add them now.

3. Blend on high until the mixture is completely smooth and creamy, which should take about 30-60 seconds. Stop and scrape down the sides if necessary to ensure everything is blended well. - If the smoothie is too thick, you can add a little more water to reach your desired consistency.

4. Taste your Beet Vitality Smoothie. If you'd like it sweeter, add a bit more honey or maple syrup and blend again. If you want a stronger ginger flavor, consider adding a little more fresh ginger and blending again. Pour the smoothie into a glass or a to-go container. Garnish with a slice of lemon or a few orange segments if desired.

TIPS:

- You can prepare the ingredients ahead of time and store them in the refrigerator for a quick smoothie when you need an energizing boost.

- For a creamier texture, consider adding a half avocado or a scoop of yogurt.

- This smoothie is not only delicious but also a fantastic way to incorporate more vegetables into your diet.

> *Enjoy your refreshing and nutrient-packed Beet Vitality Smoothie!*

Day 10: Feel the Flow

I nourish myself because I matter.

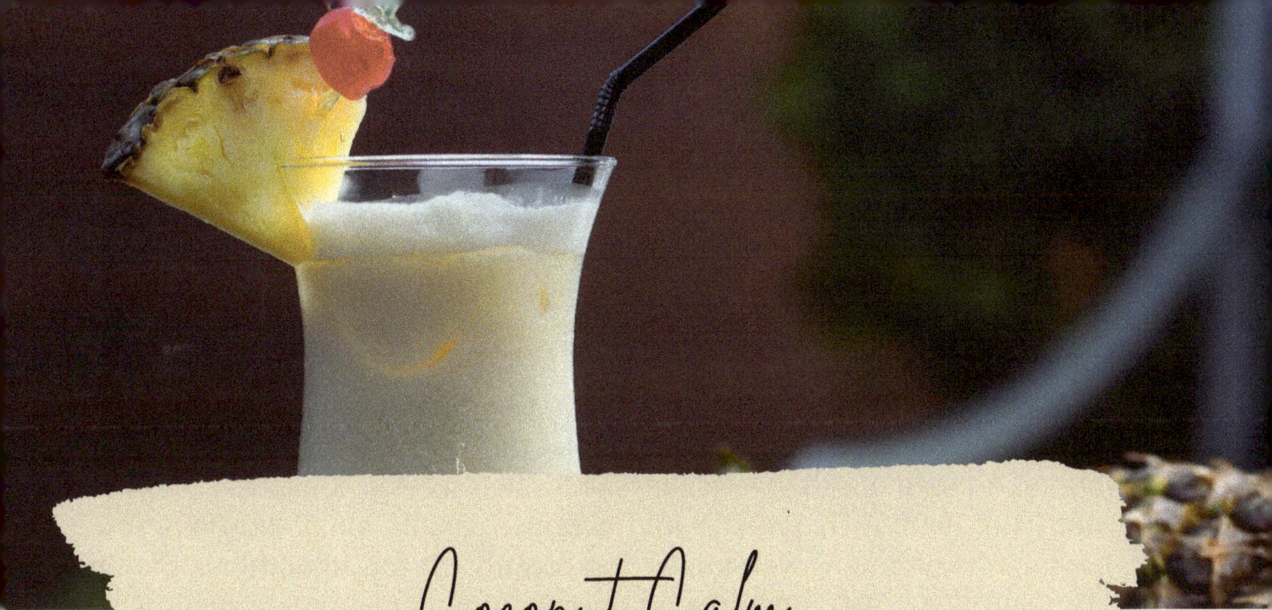

Coconut Calm

Coconut milk, pineapple, banana, chia seeds

The Coconut Calm Smoothie is a creamy, tropical treat that combines coconut milk, pineapple, and banana, enhanced with nutritious chia seeds. This delightful smoothie is not only delicious but also supports digestion and replenishes your body with essential nutrients, making it an excellent choice for breakfast or a refreshing snack.

INGREDIENTS:

- 1 cup coconut milk (canned or carton)
- 1 cup fresh or frozen pineapple chunks
- 1 medium ripe banana
- 2 tablespoons chia seeds

OPTIONAL ADD-INS:

- 1 tablespoon honey or maple syrup: For extra sweetness if desired.
- a pinch of salt: To enhance flavor and balance the sweetness.
- 1/2 teaspoon vanilla extract: For an extra layer of flavor.
- Ice cubes: For a chilled smoothie.

INSTRUCTIONS:

1. If you haven't done so already, chop the pineapple into chunks if you are using fresh pineapple. Frozen pineapple can be used directly. Peel the banana and break it into smaller pieces for more effortless blending. Measure out the coconut milk and chia seeds.

2. In a high-speed blender, add the coconut milk, pineapple chunks, banana pieces, and chia seeds. - If you're using any optional ingredients, such as honey, a pinch of salt, or ice cubes, add them at this point. Blend on high until the mixture is smooth and creamy, usually about 30-60 seconds. Ensure everything is well-mixed and creamy. If the smoothie is too thick for your liking, you can add a bit of coconut milk or water to achieve your desired consistency.

3. Taste your Coconut Calm Smoothie. If you prefer a sweeter taste, feel free to add more honey or maple syrup and blend again. If you choose a stronger coconut flavor, feel free to adjust the amount of coconut milk to your taste. Pour the smoothie into a glass or a to-go container. If desired, you can garnish with a sprinkle of chia seeds on top or a slice of pineapple on the rim.

TIPS:

- This smoothie is perfect for a post-workout recovery or as a refreshing treat on a hot day.

- Add a handful of spinach for an extra boost of nutrients without significantly altering the flavor.

- You can prepare the ingredients ahead of time and keep them in the fridge or freezer for a quick smoothie whenever you need it.

> *Enjoy the refreshing and soothing benefits of your Coconut Calm Smoothie!*

What does balance feel like today?

Day 11:
Stay *Steady*

*Radiate kindness and love;
they come back to you tenfold*

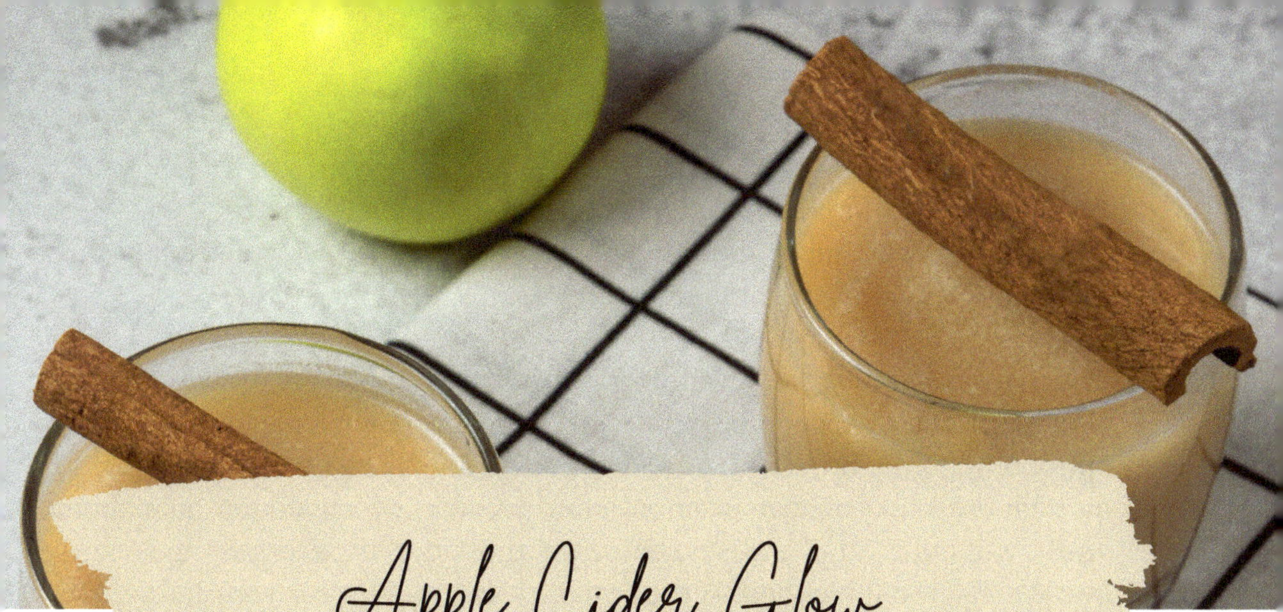

Apple Cider Glow

Green apple, cinnamon, ACV (apple cider vinegar), cucumber, water

The Apple Cider Glow Smoothie is a refreshing and invigorating drink that combines the tartness of green apple with the warming spice of cinnamon, the cleansing properties of apple cider vinegar (ACV), and the hydrating benefits of cucumber. This smoothie not only helps regulate blood sugar levels but also promotes clearer skin, making it an excellent choice for a healthy start to your day or a revitalizing afternoon pick-me-up.

INGREDIENTS:

- 1 medium green apple, cored and chopped
- 1/2 teaspoon ground cinnamon
- 1-2 tablespoons apple cider vinegar (ACV)
- 1/2 cucumber, peeled and chopped
- 1 cup filtered water

OPTIONAL ADD-INS:

- 1 tablespoon honey or maple syrup: For extra sweetness, if desired.
- 1 tablespoon chia seeds: For added fiber and omega-3 fatty acids.
- Ice cubes: For a chilled, refreshing smoothie.

INSTRUCTIONS:

1. Wash the green apple and chop it into chunks, removing the core. Peel and chop the cucumber into smaller pieces for more effortless blending. Measure out the ground cinnamon and apple cider vinegar.

2. In a high-speed blender, add the chopped green apple, cucumber, ground cinnamon, apple cider vinegar, and filtered water. If you're using any optional ingredients, such as honey or chia seeds, add them now. Blend on high until the mixture is smooth and creamy, which should take about 30-60 seconds. Stop and scrape down the sides if necessary to ensure everything is well blended. If the smoothie is too thick for your liking, you can add more filtered water to adjust the consistency.

3. Taste your Apple Cider Glow Smoothie. If you prefer a sweeter drink, feel free to add a bit more honey or maple syrup and blend again. Pour the smoothie into a glass or a to-go container. If desired, garnish with a sprinkle of cinnamon on top or a slice of green apple.

TIPS:

- For added health benefits and flavor, consider adding a handful of spinach for an extra boost of nutrients without impacting the taste.

- This smoothie is perfect for a refreshing morning drink or as an afternoon energizer.

- You can prepare your ingredients ahead of time and store them in the refrigerator to make blending quick and easy.

> *Enjoy your revitalizing and nourishing.*
> *Apple Cider Glow Smoothie!*

Day 11: Stay *Steady*

I move through this day with ease and intention.

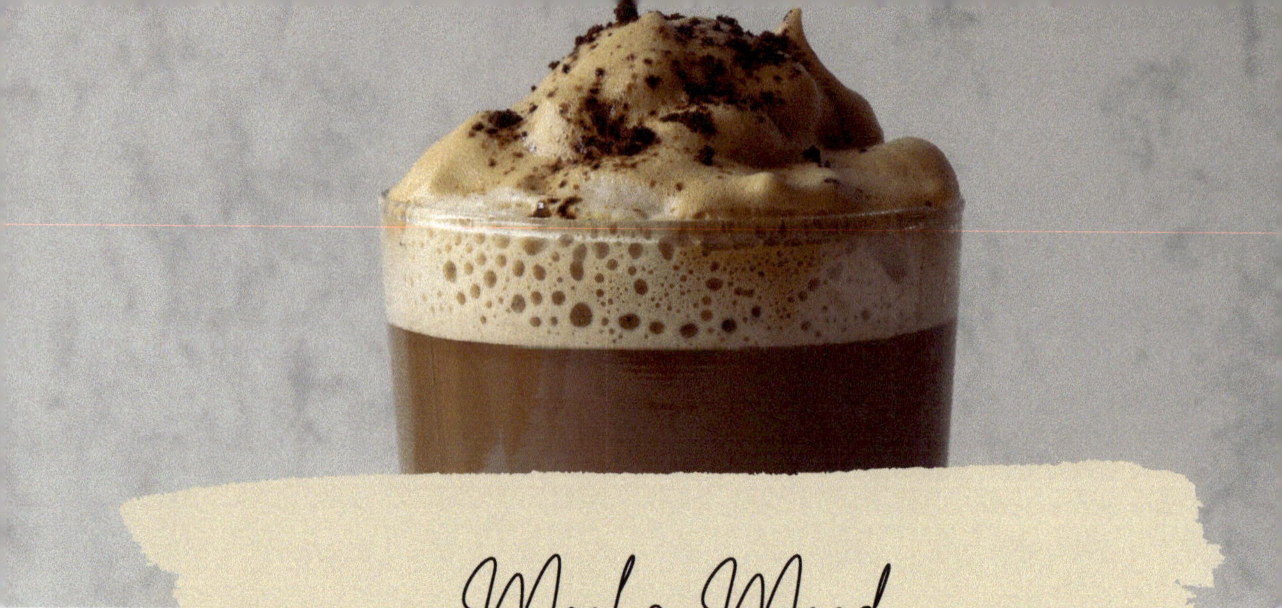

Mocha Mood

Cold brew, oat milk, cacao powder, banana, nut butter

The Mocha Mood Smoothie is a delightful blend that combines the rich flavors of cold brew coffee with creamy oat milk, cocoa powder, banana, and nut butter. This indulgent beverage serves as an excellent pick-me-up, perfect for an afternoon reset or when you need an energy boost. It's mood-lifting and satisfying, offering a delicious way to enjoy your caffeine while fueling your body with essential nutrients.

INGREDIENTS:

- 1 cup cold brew coffee
- 1 cup unsweetened oat milk
- 2 tablespoons unsweetened cacao powder
- 1 medium ripe banana
- 2 tablespoons nut butter (almond, peanut, or cashew)

OPTIONAL ADD-INS:

- 1 tablespoon maple syrup or honey: For additional sweetness if desired.
- 1/2 teaspoon vanilla extract: For an extra flavor boost.
- A pinch of sea salt: To enhance the flavors.
- Ice cubes: For a colder, frosty smoothie.

INSTRUCTIONS:

1. If you haven't already, brew your cold-brew coffee and chill it in the refrigerator. Peel the banana and cut it into chunks for more effortless blending. Measure out the oat milk, cacao powder, and nut butter.

2. In a high-speed blender, add the cold brew coffee, oat milk, cacao powder, banana, and nut butter. If you're using any optional ingredients, such as maple syrup, vanilla extract, or ice cubes, add them to the blender now. Blend on high until the mixture is smooth and creamy, about 30-60 seconds. Stop to scrape down the sides if necessary to ensure everything is well combined. If the smoothie is thicker than desired, you can add a bit of oat milk or cold brew to reach your preferred consistency.

3. Taste your Mocha Mood Smoothie. If you'd like it sweeter, add more maple syrup or honey and blend briefly. For a stronger chocolate flavor, you can add an extra tablespoon of cacao powder. Pour the smoothie into a glass or a to-go container. For an additional touch, sprinkle some cacao powder or cocoa nibs on top.

TIPS:

- This smoothie is perfect for an afternoon snack or as a quick breakfast option for a busy morning.

- You can prepare your ingredients the night before for an even quicker smoothie in the morning.

- For a fun twist, try adding a spoonful of your favorite protein powder for an extra protein boost.

> *Enjoy your delicious and energizing Mocha Mood Smoothie as a fantastic way to lift your spirits and recharge your afternoon!*

What am I beginning to see more clearly?

Day 12: Light *Up Inside*

Live authentically; your truth inspires others to do the same.

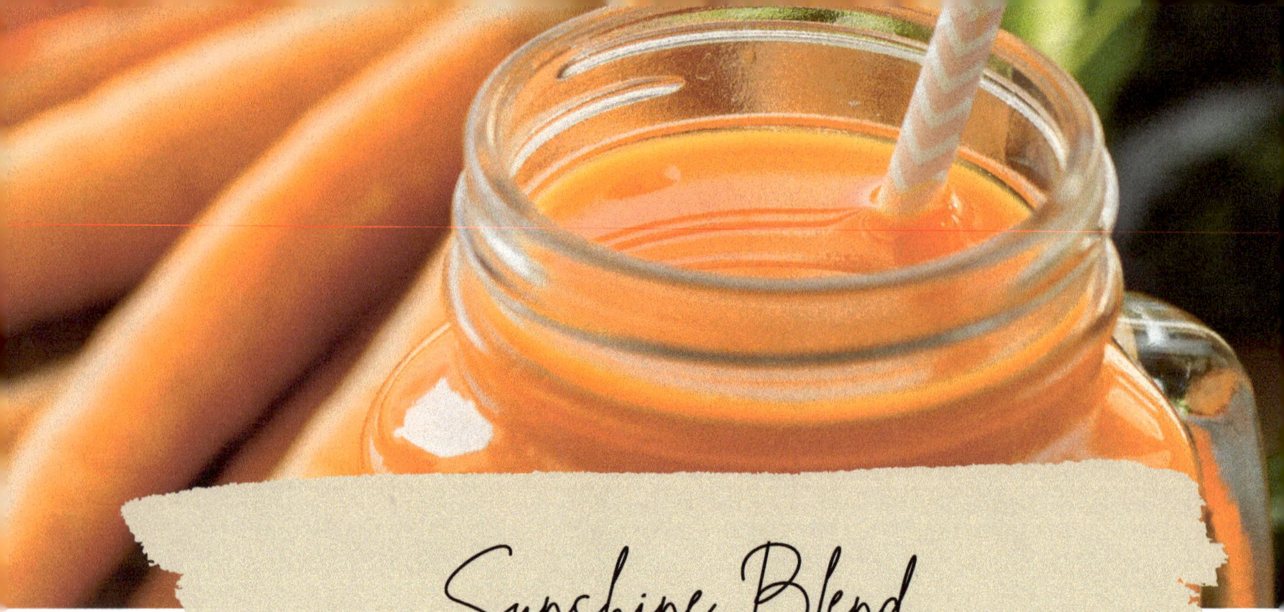

Sunshine Blend

Carrot, mango, ginger, orange juice

The Sunshine Blend Smoothie is a bright and uplifting drink that combines the natural sweetness of mango and orange juice with the earthiness of carrots and a kick of ginger. This vibrant smoothie is rich in beta-carotene, which supports skin health and adds a beautiful glow, making it an excellent choice for a nutritious start to your day or a refreshing afternoon pick-me-up.

INGREDIENTS:

- 1 medium carrot, peeled and chopped
- 1 cup ripe mango, peeled and diced
- 1-inch piece of fresh ginger, peeled
- 1 cup fresh orange juice

OPTIONAL ADD-INS:

- 1 tablespoon honey or agave syrup: For extra sweetness, if desired.
- 1 tablespoon chia seeds or flaxseeds: To boost fiber and omega-3 content.
- A handful of spinach: For added nutrients without significantly altering the flavor.
- Ice cubes: For a chilled, refreshing smoothie.

INSTRUCTIONS:

1. Peel and chop the carrot into small pieces for more effortless blending. Peel and dice the mango, removing the pit. Peel the ginger and slice it into smaller pieces for more effortless blending. Squeeze enough fresh oranges to get 1 cup of juice. Alternatively, you can use store-bought orange juice (preferably without added sugars).

2. In a high-speed blender, add the chopped carrot, diced mango, fresh ginger, and orange juice. - If you're using any optional ingredients, such as honey, chia seeds, or ice cubes, add them now. Blend on high until all ingredients are smooth and creamy, about 30-60 seconds. Stop to scrape down the sides if necessary to ensure everything is well mixed. If the smoothie is thicker than you prefer, you can add a little more orange juice or water to reach your desired consistency.

3. Taste your Sunshine Blend Smoothie. If you'd like it sweeter, you can add more honey or agave and blend again. Adjust the ginger based on your preference—add more if you want a stronger zing! Pour the smoothie into a glass or a to-go container. Garnish with a slice of mango or carrot on the rim if desired.

TIPS:

- This smoothie is fantastic for a refreshing breakfast or an energizing snack.
- You can prepare the ingredients the night before and store them in the refrigerator for a quick blend in the morning.
- Experiment by adding other fruits, such as pineapple or berries, for a different flavor profile!

> *Enjoy your radiant and nutritious Sunshine Blend Smoothie as a delicious way to nourish your skin and brighten your day!*

Day 12: Light Up Inside

My power is rooted in presence.

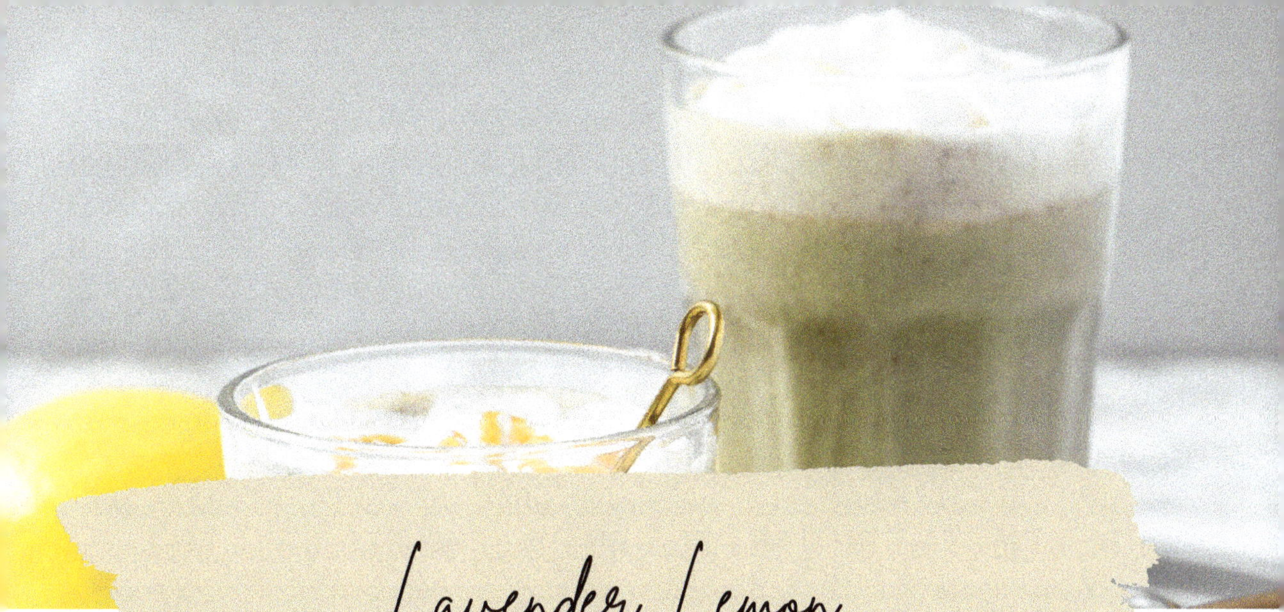

Lavender Lemon

Lemon, unsweetened almond milk, a touch of lavender (optional), vanilla

Lavender Lemon Smoothie is a refreshing and soothing drink that combines the zesty brightness of lemon with the creamy texture of unsweetened almond milk and a subtle hint of lavender. This delightful smoothie is cooling and calming, making it an excellent choice for a relaxing afternoon treat or a gentle start to your morning.

INGREDIENTS:

- 1 large lemon, juiced
- 1 cup unsweetened almond milk
- 1-2 teaspoons dried culinary lavender (optional)
- 1/2 teaspoon vanilla extract
- 1 tablespoon honey or maple syrup

INSTRUCTIONS:

1. Juice the lemon, making sure to strain out any seeds. Measure out the almond milk, vanilla extract, and lavender. If you're using dried lavender, make sure it is food-grade and suitable for consumption.

2. In a high-speed blender, add the lemon juice, unsweetened almond milk, dried lavender (if using), vanilla extract, and honey or maple syrup. If you prefer a chilled smoothie, feel free to add a handful of ice cubes. Blend on high for 30-60 seconds or until the mixture is smooth and well combined. If using lavender, you may want to blend for a more extended period to help break down the petals and infuse the flavor.

3. Taste your Lavender Lemon Smoothie. If you'd like it sweeter, add more honey or maple syrup and blend again. If the lavender flavor is too strong or if you want more lemon brightness, adjust accordingly by adding more lemon juice or a pinch more lavender. Pour the smoothie into a glass or a to-go container. For a decorative touch, you can garnish with a sprig of fresh lavender or a lemon slice on the rim.

TIPS:

- This smoothie is perfect for a refreshing afternoon pick-me-up or a relaxing evening treat.

- You can adjust the lavender intensity according to your taste by starting with a small amount.

- Consider adding a handful of spinach or kale for added nutrients without significantly changing the flavor.

> *Enjoy your calming and refreshing Lavender Lemon Smoothie!*

Where do I feel most alive in my body?

“

Day 13: Strong & Soft

Every challenge is an opportunity to reveal your strength.

”

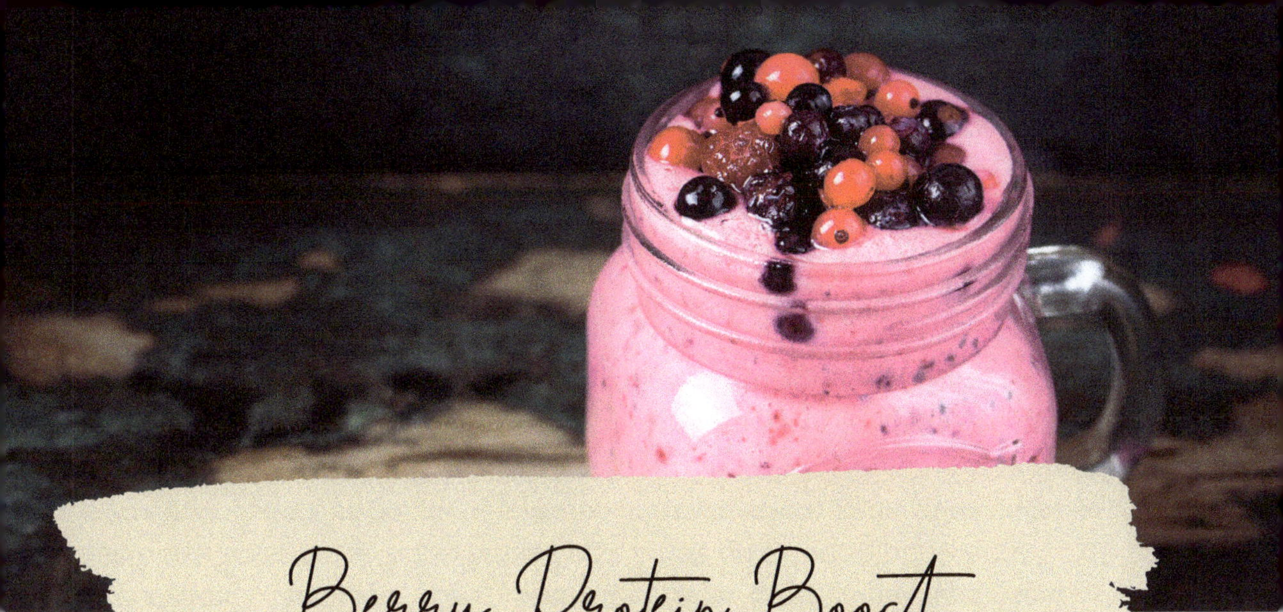

Berry Protein Boost

Mixed berries, almond milk, flaxseed, vanilla protein (optional)

The Berry Protein Boost Smoothie is a delicious and nutrient-dense drink that combines the natural sweetness of mixed berries with creamy almond milk and a nutritional punch from flaxseed and optional protein powder. This smoothie is perfect for post-workout replenishment or as a nutritious breakfast option that supports strength and gut health.

INGREDIENTS:

- 1 cup mixed berries (fresh or frozen)
- 1 cup unsweetened almond milk
- 2 tablespoons ground flaxseed
- 1 scoop vanilla protein powder (optional)

OPTIONAL ADD-INS:

- 1 tablespoon honey or maple syrup: For added sweetness, if desired.
- 1/2 banana: For extra creaminess and natural sweetness.
- A handful of spinach: For added nutrients without significantly altering the flavor.
- Ice cubes: If you prefer a colder and thicker smoothie.

INSTRUCTIONS:

1. If using fresh berries, wash them thoroughly to remove any dirt or debris. If using frozen, they can be added directly to the blender. Measure out the almond milk and flaxseed. If using protein powder, have that ready to add.

2. In a high-speed blender, add the mixed berries, unsweetened almond milk, ground flaxseed, and vanilla protein powder (if using). If you're using any optional ingredients, such as honey or ice cubes, add them at this point. Blend on high until the mixture is completely smooth and creamy, about 30 to 60 seconds. Stop and scrape down the sides if necessary to ensure everything is well combined. - If the smoothie is too thick, you can add a little more almond milk or water to reach your desired consistency.

3. Taste your Berry Protein Boost Smoothie. If you'd like it sweeter, consider adding more honey or maple syrup and blending again. Adjust the protein powder according to your dietary needs and taste preferences. Pour the smoothie into a glass or a to-go container. For a decorative touch, you can garnish with a few whole berries on top.

TIPS:

- This smoothie is excellent for breakfast, a post-workout snack, or a quick meal replacement.

- Feel free to experiment with different combinations of berries or add other fruits to customize the flavor to your liking.

- You can also prepare ingredients the night before for a quick blend in the morning.

> *Enjoy your Berry Protein Boost Smoothie as a tasty way to support your fitness goals and gut health!*

Day 13:
Strong & Soft

I give myself permission to unplug and replenish.

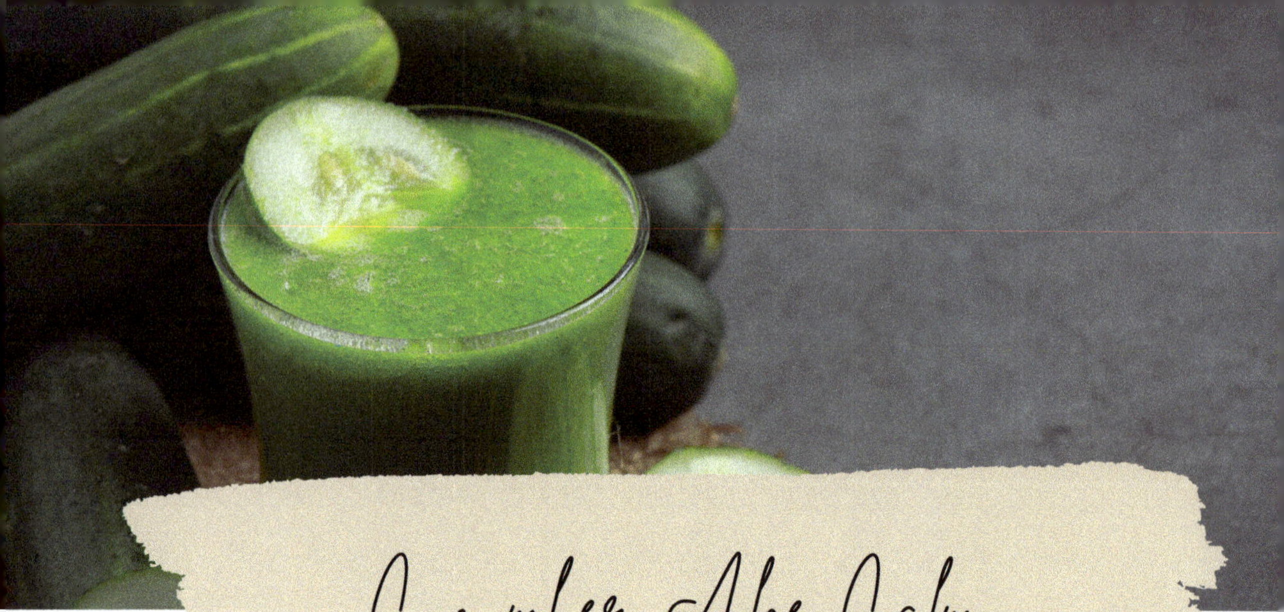

Cucumber Aloe Calm

Cucumber, aloe juice, pear, mint

The Cucumber Aloe Calm Smoothie is a refreshing and hydrating drink designed to soothe your digestive system and promote overall wellness. This gentle blend of cucumber, aloe juice, ripe pear, and fresh mint creates a light and cooling smoothie, perfect for hot days or when you need a refreshing treat.

INGREDIENTS:

- 1 medium cucumber, peeled and chopped:
- 1/2 cup aloe
- 1 ripe pear, cored and chopped
- 1/4 cup fresh mint leaves

OPTIONAL ADD-INS:

- 1 tablespoon honey or agave syrup: For extra sweetness, if desired.
- 1 tablespoon chia seeds: For added fiber and omega-3 fatty acids.
- Juice of 1 lime: For a zesty kick and an additional layer of flavor.
- Ice cubes: If you prefer a chilled smoothie.

INSTRUCTIONS:

1. Peel and chop the cucumber into smaller pieces for more effortless blending. Core and chop the pear into chunks. Measure out the aloe juice and wash the mint leaves.

2. In a high-speed blender, combine the chopped cucumber, aloe juice, pear pieces, and fresh mint leaves. If using optional ingredients like honey, lime juice, chia seeds, or ice cubes, add them now. Blend on high until smooth and creamy, which should take about 30-60 seconds. Stop and scrape down the sides if necessary to ensure all ingredients are well blended. If the smoothie is too thick, add a little more aloe juice or water to reach your desired consistency.

3. Taste your Cucumber Aloe Calm Smoothie. If you'd like it sweeter, add more honey or agave syrup and blend again. If you prefer a stronger mint flavor, you can add a few more mint leaves and blend again. Pour the smoothie into a glass or a to-go container. If desired, garnish with a slice of cucumber or a sprig of mint on top.

TIPS:

- This smoothie is perfect for a light breakfast, a post-workout refreshment, or as a soothing snack any time of the day.

- Feel free to experiment by adding other mild ingredients, such as spinach or kale, for added nutrients without compromising the flavor.

- You can prepare the ingredients ahead of time and store them in the refrigerator for a quick blend.

> *Enjoy your refreshing and soothing.*
> *Cucumber Aloe Calm Smoothie!*

Have I trusted myself this week? Why? Why not?

Day 14: Recharge & Reflect

Trust the process; growth comes from discomfort.

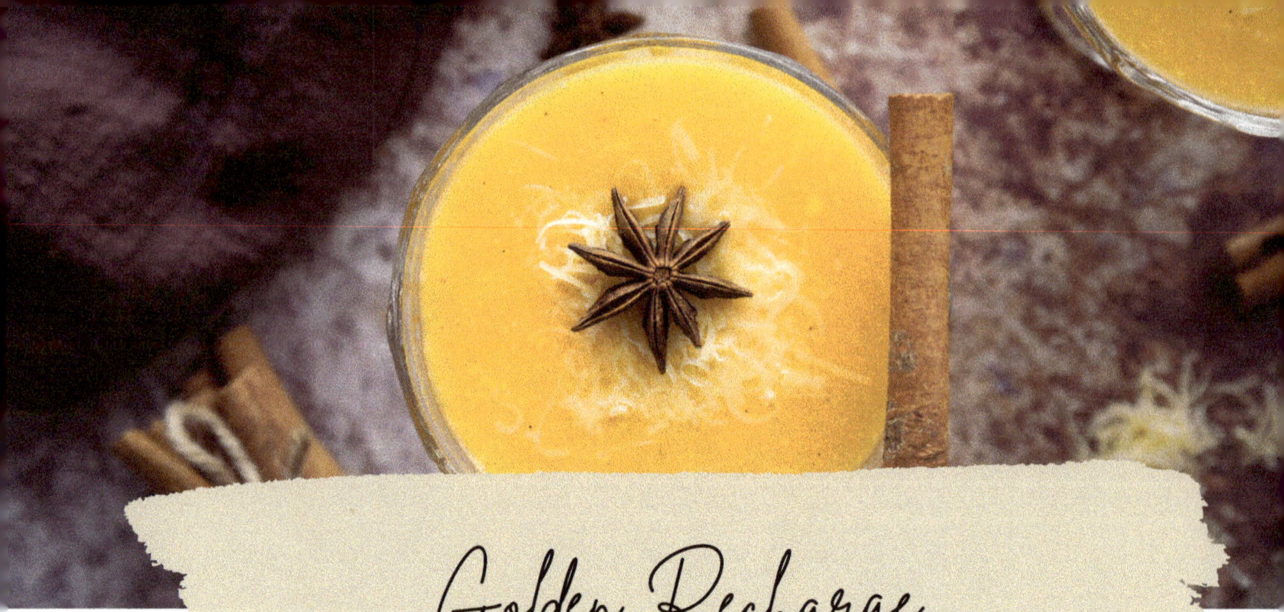

Golden Recharge

Turmeric, banana, oat milk, cinnamon, honey

The Golden Recharge Smoothie is a warming and nourishing drink that combines the powerful anti-inflammatory benefits of turmeric with the creamy sweetness of banana, the smoothness of oat milk, and the warmth of cinnamon. This delightful smoothie is perfect for an energizing breakfast or a comforting afternoon boost.

INGREDIENTS:

- 1 medium banana
- 1 cup unsweetened oat milk
- 1 teaspoon ground turmeric
- 1/2 teaspoon ground cinnamon
- 1 tablespoon honey

OPTIONAL ADD-INS:

- 1 tablespoon chia seeds or flaxseeds: For added fiber and omega-3 fatty acids.
- A pinch of black pepper: To enhance the absorption of turmeric's active compound, curcumin.
- A handful of spinach: For extra nutrients without significantly altering the flavor.
- Ice cubes: If you prefer a colder smoothie.

INSTRUCTIONS:

1. Peel the banana and break it into chunks for more effortless blending. - Measure out the oat milk, turmeric, cinnamon, and honey.

2. In a high-speed blender, add the banana, oat milk, ground turmeric, ground cinnamon, and honey. If you're using any optional ingredients, such as chia seeds, black pepper, or ice cubes, add them now. Blend on high until the mixture is smooth and creamy, usually about 30-60 seconds. Stop and scrape down the sides if necessary to ensure everything is well combined. If the smoothie is too thick for your liking, add a little more oat milk to reach your desired consistency.

3. Taste your Golden Recharge Smoothie. If you'd like it sweeter, add more honey or maple syrup and blend briefly. You can adjust the turmeric and cinnamon based on your flavor preference. Pour the smoothie into a glass or a to-go container. For garnish, you can sprinkle a little extra cinnamon on top or add a slice of banana.

TIPS:

- This smoothie is perfect for a warming breakfast or a mid-afternoon pick-me-up.

- Feel free to experiment with different spices, such as nutmeg or ginger, for a unique flavor twist.

- Preparing the ingredients in advance can make for a quick and easy smoothie option when you're on the go.

> *Enjoy your delicious and nourishing Golden Recharge Smoothie, packed with health benefits and great flavor!*

"

Day 14: Recharge & Reflect

The more I honor my needs, the more I glow.

"

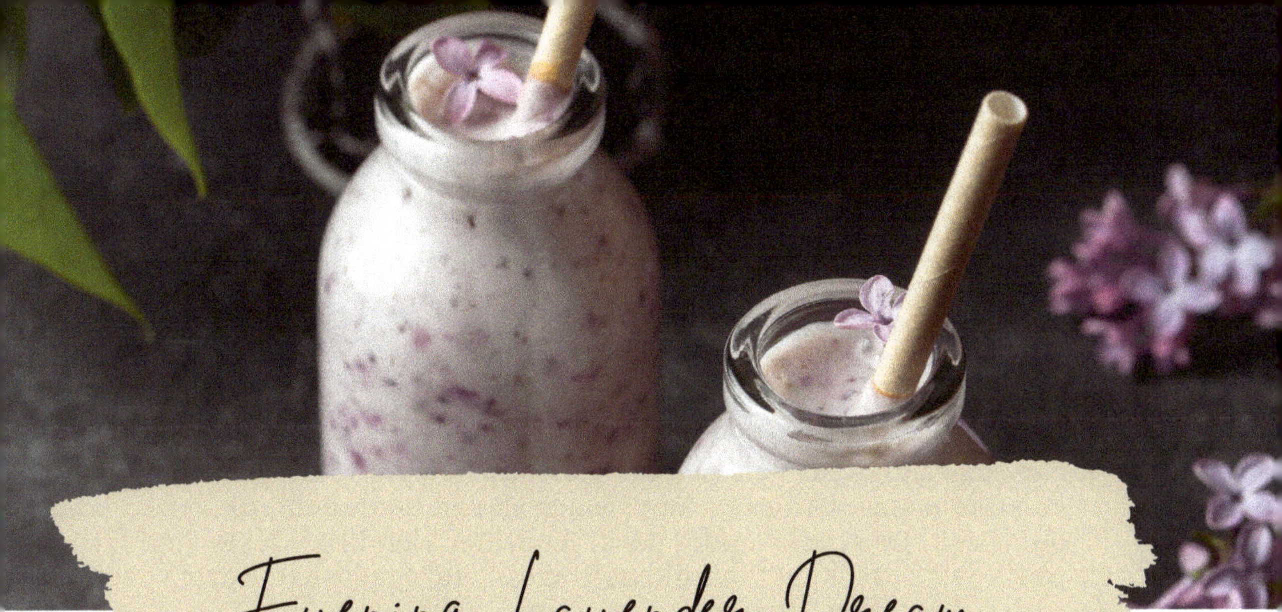

Evening Lavender Dream

Warm almond milk, lavender, date, cinnamon

The Evening Lavender Dream Smoothie is a warm and soothing blend designed to help you unwind and relax before bedtime. Combining the calming properties of lavender with sweet dates, aromatic cinnamon, and creamy almond milk, this delightful smoothie is perfect for promoting restful sleep and a peaceful evening routine.

INGREDIENTS:

- 1 cup warm almond milk
- 1 teaspoon dried culinary lavender
- 2-3 Medjool dates (pitted)
- 1/2 teaspoon ground cinnamon

OPTIONAL ADD-INS:

- A pinch of sea salt: To enhance the flavors and balance sweetness.
- 1/2 teaspoon vanilla extract: For extra flavor depth.
- 1 tablespoon chia seeds: For added fiber and omega-3 fatty acids.
- Ice cubes: If you prefer a chilled version (though warm is recommended for bedtime).

INSTRUCTIONS:

1. Measure out the almond milk and lavender. If you're using whole dates, ensure they're pitted and chop them into smaller pieces for more effortless blending. In a small saucepan, gently heat the almond milk over low heat until warm but not boiling. Alternatively, you can heat it in the microwave for about 30-60 seconds.

2. In a high-speed blender, combine the warm almond milk, dried lavender, chopped dates, and ground cinnamon. If you're using optional ingredients like sea salt, vanilla extract, or chia seeds, add them now. Blend on high until the mixture is smooth and creamy, which should take about 30-45 seconds. If you want a stronger lavender flavor, consider blending a bit longer. If the smoothie is too thick for your liking, you can add a splash of warm water or almond milk until you achieve your desired consistency.

3. Taste your Evening Lavender Dream Smoothie. If you prefer a sweeter taste, you can add more dates or a hint of honey and blend again. If you'd like a more pronounced cinnamon flavor, feel free to add a little more cinnamon and blend. Pour the smoothie into a cozy mug or a glass. For a decorative touch, consider garnishing with a sprinkle of cinnamon or a few lavender buds on top. Enjoy it warm to promote relaxation and a calm evening ambiance!

TIPS:

- This smoothie is perfect for winding down after a long day. Enjoy it as part of your nighttime routine.

- Consider making a larger batch and storing it in the fridge if you want to prepare it in advance.

- Warm it before consuming it for optimal results.

- Feel free to experiment with other calming herbs (like chamomile) if you want to change the flavor profile.

> *Indulge in the soothing and aromatic experience of your Evening Lavender Dream Smoothie and enjoy a peaceful night's sleep!*

What is one win from this week?

Recharge & *Nourish Check-in*

> *Refuel, find flow, and restore energy and rhythm.*

I am a Divine Original

What did I learn about my energy this week? What habits or boundaries helped me feel more sustained, and where am I still feeling depleted? How will I honor my energy moving forward?

Day 15: Ground & Breath

Surround yourself with positivity, and watch your light shine brighter

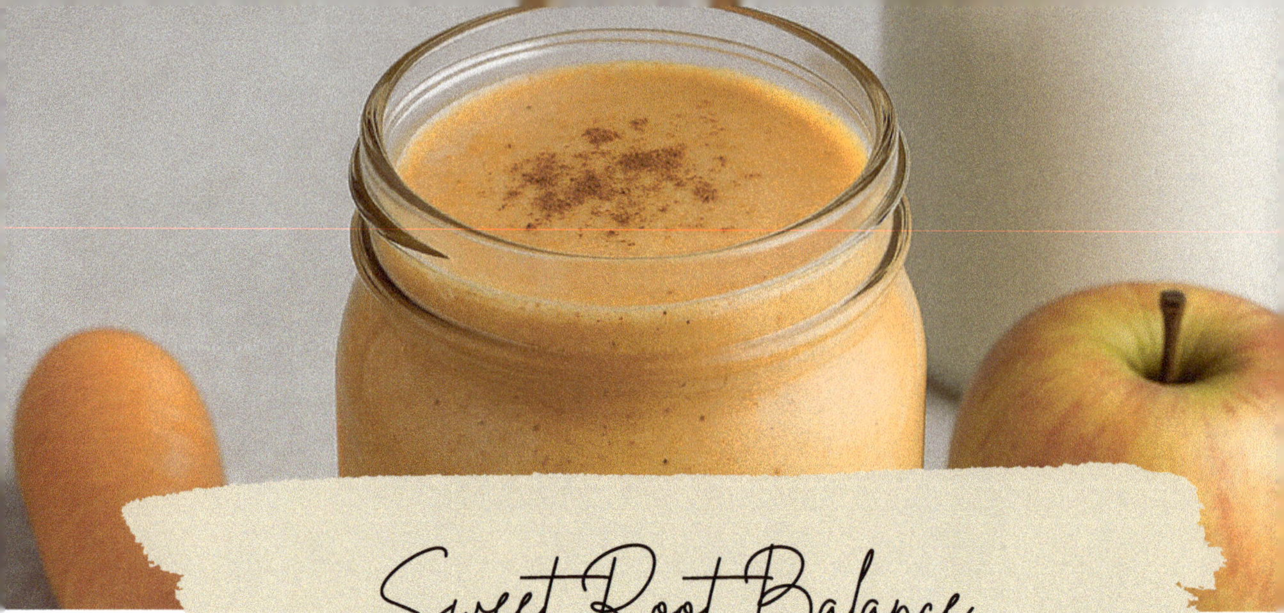

Sweet Root Balance

Carrot, apple, ginger, cinnamon, almond milk

The Sweet Root Balance Smoothie is a nourishing and grounding beverage that combines the natural sweetness of carrots and apples with the warming spice of ginger and cinnamon. Enhanced with creamy almond milk, this smoothie is packed with nutrients that support hormonal balance, making it an ideal choice for breakfast or a midday snack.

INGREDIENTS:

- 1 medium carrot, peeled and chopped
- 1 medium apple (any variety), cored and chopped
- 1-inch piece of fresh ginger, peeled and grated
- ½ teaspoon ground cinnamon
- 1 cup unsweetened almond milk

OPTIONAL ADD-INS:

- 1 tablespoon chia seeds or flaxseed for added fiber and omega-3 fatty acids.
- 1 tablespoon maple syrup or honey if you prefer a sweeter taste.
- ½ banana for additional creaminess and natural sweetness.
- Ice cubes for a colder smoothie.

INSTRUCTIONS:

1. Peel and chop the carrot into smaller pieces for more effortless blending. Core the apple and cut it into pieces (you can keep the skin on for extra fiber). Peel and grate the ginger for easy blending. Measure out the almond milk and any optional ingredients you plan to use.

2. In a high-speed blender, combine the chopped carrot, apple pieces, grated ginger, ground cinnamon, and almond milk. If you're using any optional ingredients like chia seeds, honey, or ice cubes, add them at this stage. Blend on high speed until the mixture is completely smooth and creamy, about 30 to 60 seconds. Make sure to scrape down the sides to ensure all ingredients are well blended. If the smoothie is too thick for your liking, you can add a little more almond milk to reach your desired consistency.

3. Taste your Sweet Root Balance Smoothie. If you want it sweeter, add a bit more honey or maple syrup and blend again. Adjust the ginger and cinnamon according to your taste preference for a stronger flavor profile. Pour the smoothie into a glass or a to-go container. You can garnish with a sprinkle of cinnamon or serve with a slice of apple on the rim if desired.

TIPS:

- This smoothie is an excellent option for grounding yourself during busy days or as a comforting evening treat.

- You can prepare the ingredients in advance and store them in the refrigerator for a quick and easy blend whenever you need it.

- Feel free to experiment with other spices, such as nutmeg or cardamom, for added flavor variety.

> *Enjoy your nourishing and hormone-supportive Sweet Root Balance Smoothie!*

Day 15: Ground & Breath

Healing is not linear—but it is mine.

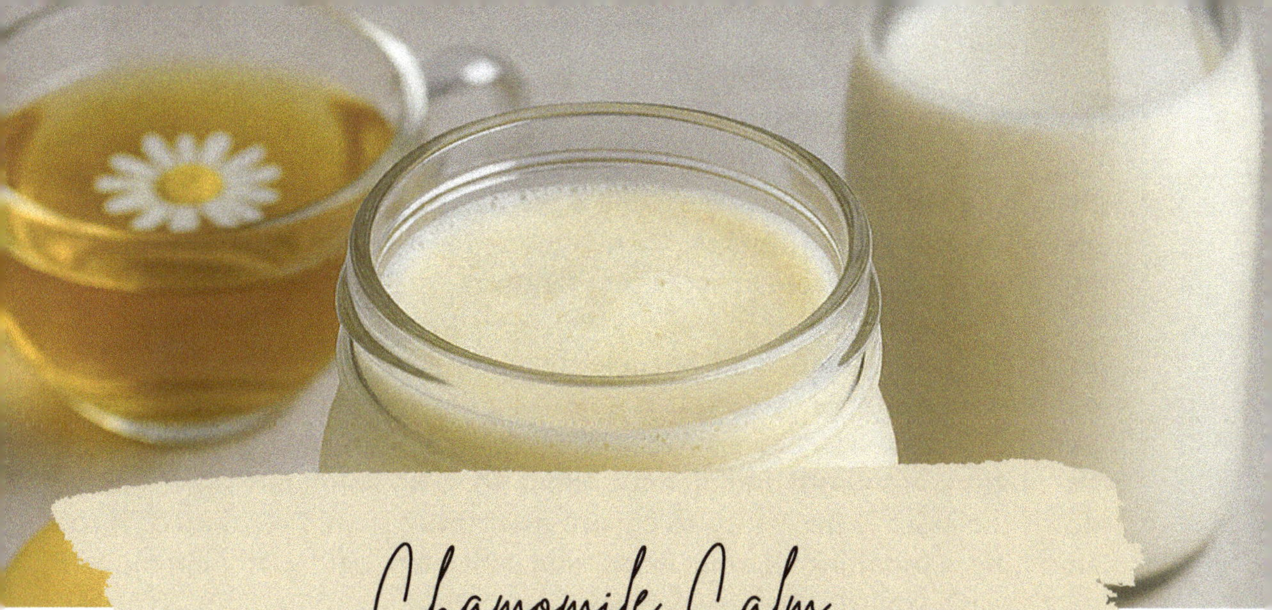

Chamomile Calm

Brewed chamomile tea (cooled), banana, oat milk, vanilla

Chamomile Calm is a soothing and comforting drink designed to help you unwind and prepare for a restful night's sleep. Combining brewed chamomile tea with the natural sweetness of banana, creamy oat milk, and a hint of vanilla, this smoothie is perfect for easing tension and promoting relaxation. It's a delightful way to enjoy the calming properties of chamomile.

INGREDIENTS:

- 1 cup brewed chamomile tea (cooled)
- 1 ripe banana
- 1 cup unsweetened oat milk
- ½ teaspoon vanilla extract

OPTIONAL ADD-INS:

- 1 tablespoon honey or maple syrup: For a sweeter taste.
- 1 tablespoon chia seeds: For added fiber and omega-3 fatty acids.
- A pinch of cinnamon: To enhance the flavor and add warmth. - Ice cubes: For a chilled, refreshing smoothie.

INSTRUCTIONS:

1. Brew a cup of chamomile tea using a tea bag or loose flowers. Allow it to steep for about 5-7 minutes, then remove the tea bag or strain out the flowers. Let the tea cool to room temperature.

2. In a high-speed blender, add the cooled chamomile tea, banana, unsweetened oat milk, and vanilla extract. If you're using any optional ingredients, such as honey, chia seeds, or ice cubes, add them now. Blend on high speed until the mixture is smooth and creamy, about 30 to 45 seconds. Stop to scrape down the sides if necessary to ensure everything is well combined. If the smoothie is too thick for your liking, add a bit more oat milk or chamomile tea to reach your desired consistency.

3. Taste your Chamomile Calm Smoothie. If you'd like it sweeter, you can add more honey or maple syrup and blend again. For a stronger vanilla flavor, you can add a touch more vanilla extract. Pour the smoothie into a glass or a cozy mug. For an optional garnish, sprinkle a little cinnamon on top. Enjoy immediately to experience its comforting and soothing effects.

TIPS:

- Enjoy this smoothie as part of your evening routine to promote relaxation before bed.

- You can prepare the chamomile tea in advance and place it in the refrigerator for a quick smoothie later.

- For added variety, consider blending in a small handful of spinach for extra nutrients without significantly altering the flavor.

> *Enjoy a calming and restful afternoon or evening with your smoothie: Chamomile Calm, a delightful way to unwind at the end of the day!*

What does wellness mean to you today?

“

Day 16: Release & Rest

Wellness is about balance, honor your mind, body, and spirit equally

”

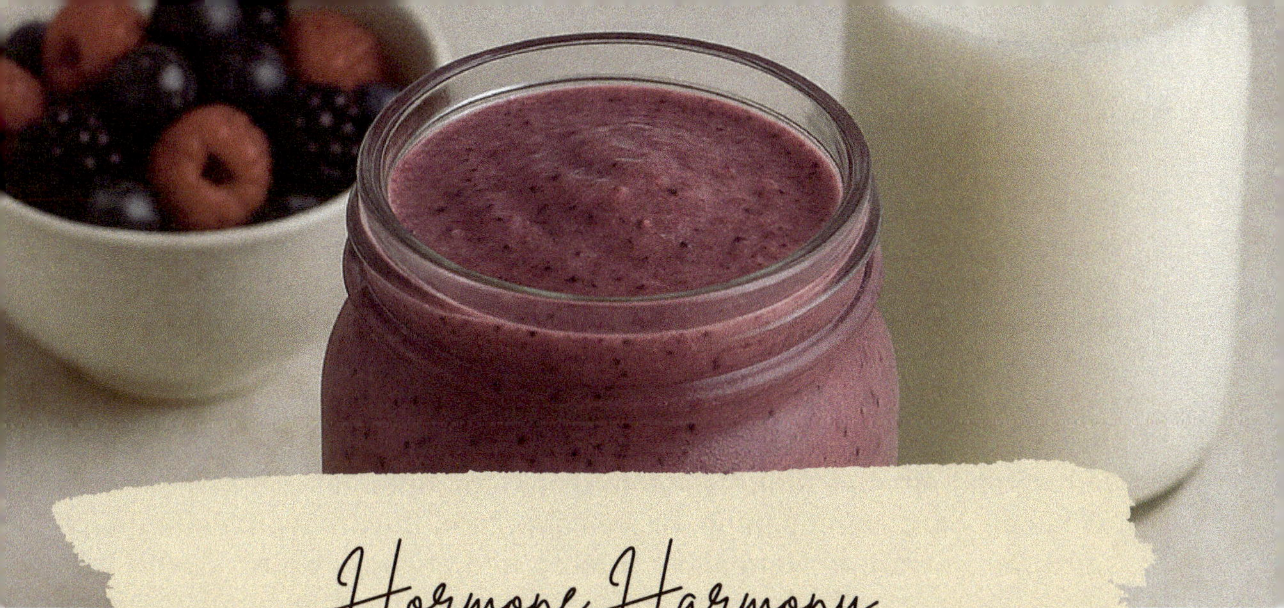

Hormone Harmony

Berries, flaxseed, almond butter, almond milk

Hormone Harmony Smoothie is a delicious and nutrient-dense blend designed to support hormonal balance in your body. Combining antioxidant-rich berries, fiber-filled flaxseeds, creamy almond butter, and nourishing almond milk, this smoothie is a fantastic option for breakfast or a mid-day snack. It offers a balance of healthy fats, fiber, and vitamins that can help stabilize mood and energy levels.

INGREDIENTS:

- 1 cup mixed berries (fresh or frozen)
- 2 tablespoons ground flaxseed
- 2 tablespoons almond butter
- 1 cup unsweetened almond milk

OPTIONAL ADD-INS:

- 1 tablespoon honey or maple syrup: For added sweetness, if desired.
- ½ ripe banana: For additional creaminess and natural sweetness.
- A pinch of cinnamon: For flavor and to help regulate blood sugar levels.
- Ice cubes: For a colder, thicker smoothie.

INSTRUCTIONS:

1. Measure out the mixed berries. If using fresh berries, rinse them thoroughly to remove any dirt or debris. If using frozen berries, you can add them directly to the blender. Have the ground flaxseed and almond butter ready. Measure out the almond milk and any optional ingredients you want to include.

2. In a high-speed blender, add the mixed berries, ground flaxseed, almond butter, and almond milk. If you're using any optional ingredients, such as honey, banana, cinnamon, or ice cubes, add them now. Blend on high until the mixture is completely smooth and creamy, which should take about 30-60 seconds. Stop and scrape down the sides if necessary to ensure everything is well-mixed. If the smoothie is too thick for your liking, you can add a little more almond milk to reach your desired consistency.

3. Taste your Hormone Harmony Smoothie. If you'd like it sweeter, add more honey or maple syrup and blend again. Adjust the amount of cinnamon or almond butter based on your preference for flavor and creaminess. Pour the smoothie into a glass or a to-go container. For an optional garnish, you can sprinkle a few extra berries or a dash of flaxseed on top. Enjoy immediately for the best flavor and nutritional benefits!

TIPS:

- This smoothie is ideally suited for quick breakfasts or as a healthy snack to keep you energized throughout the day.

- You can customize the smoothie by adding other ingredients, such as spinach, for extra nutrients without significantly altering the taste.

- Preparing ingredients ahead of time can make for a quick and convenient smoothie on busy mornings.

> *Enjoy your nourishing and hormone-balancing Hormone Harmony Smoothie!*

Day 16:
Release & Rest

I am worthy of softness, even now.

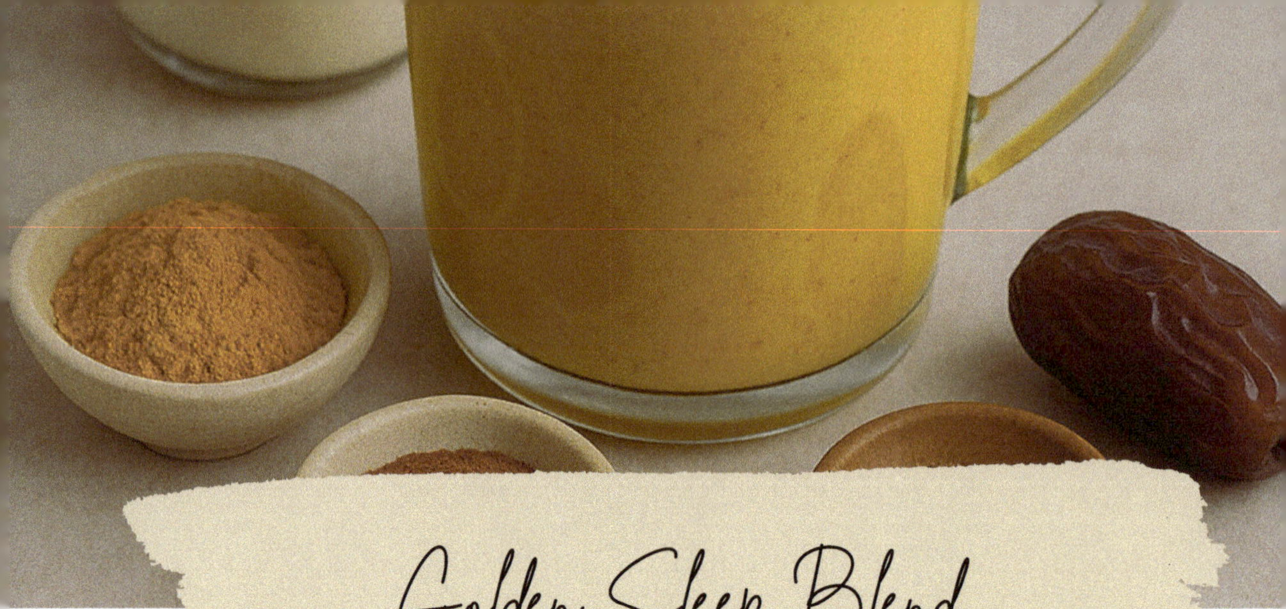

Golden Sleep Blend

Warm oat milk, turmeric, cinnamon, date, nutmeg

Golden Sleep Blend is a warm, soothing drink designed to help you unwind and prepare for restful sleep. This comforting blend of warm oat milk, turmeric, cinnamon, dates, and nutmeg is not only delicious but also packed with anti-inflammatory properties. It's perfect for a late-night treat or as part of your bedtime routine.

INGREDIENTS:

- 1 cup warm oat milk
- 1 teaspoon ground turmeric
- ½ teaspoon ground cinnamon
- 1-2 Medjool dates, pitted
- A pinch of ground nutmeg

OPTIONAL ADD-INS:

- A pinch of black pepper: Enhances the absorption of turmeric's active compound, curcumin.
- 1/4 teaspoon vanilla extract: For extra flavor depth.
- 1 tablespoon chia seeds or flaxseeds: For added fiber and omega-3 fatty acids.

INSTRUCTIONS:

1. If using whole dates, pit them and chop them into smaller pieces for easier blending. Measure out the oat milk, turmeric, cinnamon, nutmeg, and any optional ingredients as needed. - In a small saucepan, gently warm the oat milk over low heat until it's warm but not boiling. Alternatively, you can microwave it for about 30-60 seconds.

2. In a high-speed blender, combine the warm oat milk, ground turmeric, ground cinnamon, chopped dates, and a pinch of nutmeg. If you're adding any optional ingredients (such as black pepper or vanilla extract), include them at this stage.

3. Blend on high until the mixture is smooth and creamy, about 30-60 seconds. If needed, stop to scrape down the sides to ensure everything is well combined.

4. Taste your Golden Sleep Blend. If you'd like it sweeter, you can add more dates or a drizzle of honey and blend again. - Adjust the spices to your taste preference (add more nutmeg or cinnamon if desired). Pour the Golden Sleep Blend into a cozy mug. For an optional garnish, sprinkle a little extra cinnamon or nutmeg on top. Enjoy warm as part of your bedtime routine for a peaceful night's sleep.

TIPS:

- This warm drink is perfect for winding down in the evening.
- Consider incorporating it into your nighttime routine.
- You can prepare a larger batch and store it in the refrigerator, then warm individual servings as needed.
- To make it even creamier, consider adding a splash of coconut cream or other dairy-free milk alternatives.

> *Enjoy your soothing and anti-inflammatory Golden Sleep Blend as you prepare for a restful night's sleep!*

What does wellness mean to you today?

Day 17:
Nourish *Deeply*

Create a life that reflects your values and passions.

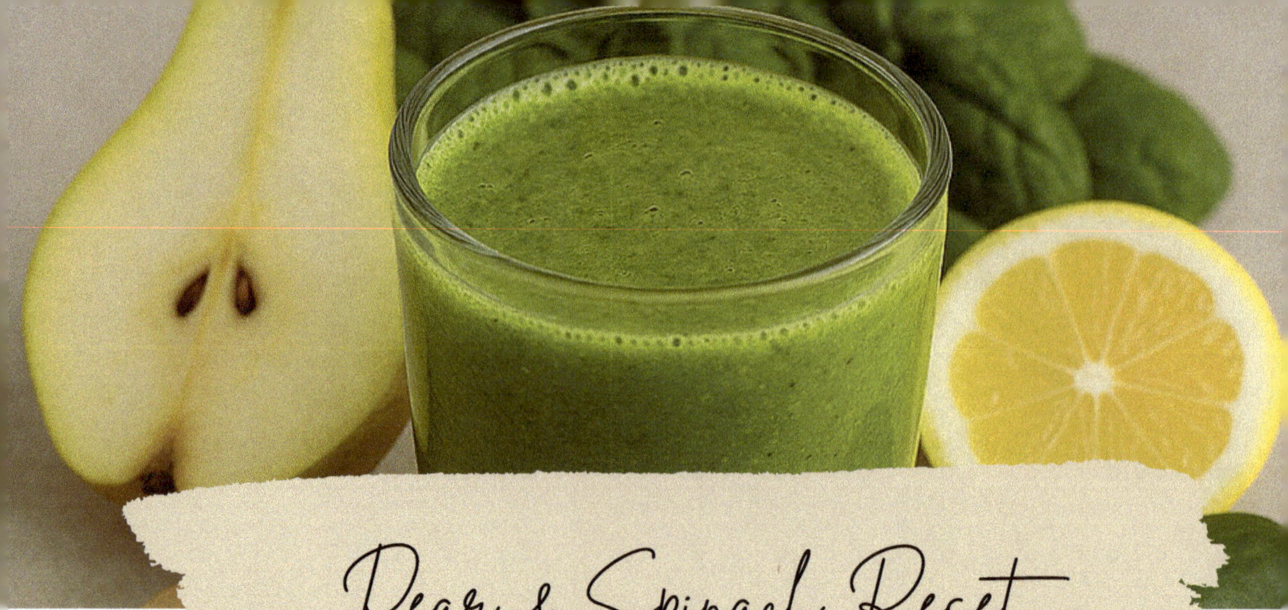

Pear & Spinach Reset

Pear, spinach, ginger, lemon, cucumber

Pear & Spinach Reset Smoothie is a refreshing and nutritious blend that combines the sweet flavor of pear with the wholesome benefits of spinach, ginger, lemon, and cucumber. This detoxifying smoothie is alkalizing and packed with vitamins and antioxidants, making it an ideal choice for promoting gut health and enhancing skin vitality.

INGREDIENTS:

- 1 ripe pear, cored and chopped
- 2 cups fresh spinach
- 1-inch piece of fresh ginger, peeled and grated
- Juice of 1 lemon
- 1/2 cucumber, peeled and chopped

OPTIONAL ADD-INS:

- 1 tablespoon chia seeds or flaxseeds: For added fiber and healthy fats.
- 1 tablespoon honey or maple syrup: For a sweeter taste.
- Ice cubes: For a chilled smoothie.

INSTRUCTIONS:

1. Wash and chop the pear, removing the core. Rinse the spinach thoroughly and remove any tough stems. Peel and grate the ginger root. Cut the lemon in half and squeeze out the juice, discarding any seeds. Peel and chop the cucumber.

2. In a high-speed blender, add the chopped pear, fresh spinach, grated ginger, lemon juice, and cucumber. If using optional ingredients like chia seeds, honey, or ice cubes, add them at this stage. Blend on high speed until the mixture is smooth and creamy, about 30 to 60 seconds. You might need to stop and scrape down the sides to ensure everything is well combined. If the smoothie is too thick for your liking, you can add a little more water or cucumber to achieve your desired consistency.

3. Taste your Pear & Spinach Reset Smoothie. If you'd like it sweeter, feel free to add more honey or maple syrup and blend again. - Adjust the ginger to your taste preference for a stronger flavor, if desired. Pour the smoothie into a glass or a to-go container. Garnish with a slice of pear or a cucumber slice on the rim if desired.

4. Enjoy immediately to maximize flavor and nutritional benefits!

TIPS:

- This smoothie is perfect as a refreshing breakfast option or a revitalizing snack at any time of the day.

- You can adjust the ingredients based on what you have on hand; other leafy greens, such as kale, can be substituted for spinach.

- Consider making a larger batch and storing it in the refrigerator, but it's best to consume it fresh for optimal health benefits.

> *Enjoy your refreshing and nourishing Pear & Spinach Reset Smoothie!*

Day 17: Nourish *Deeply*

Balance is a gift I give myself daily.

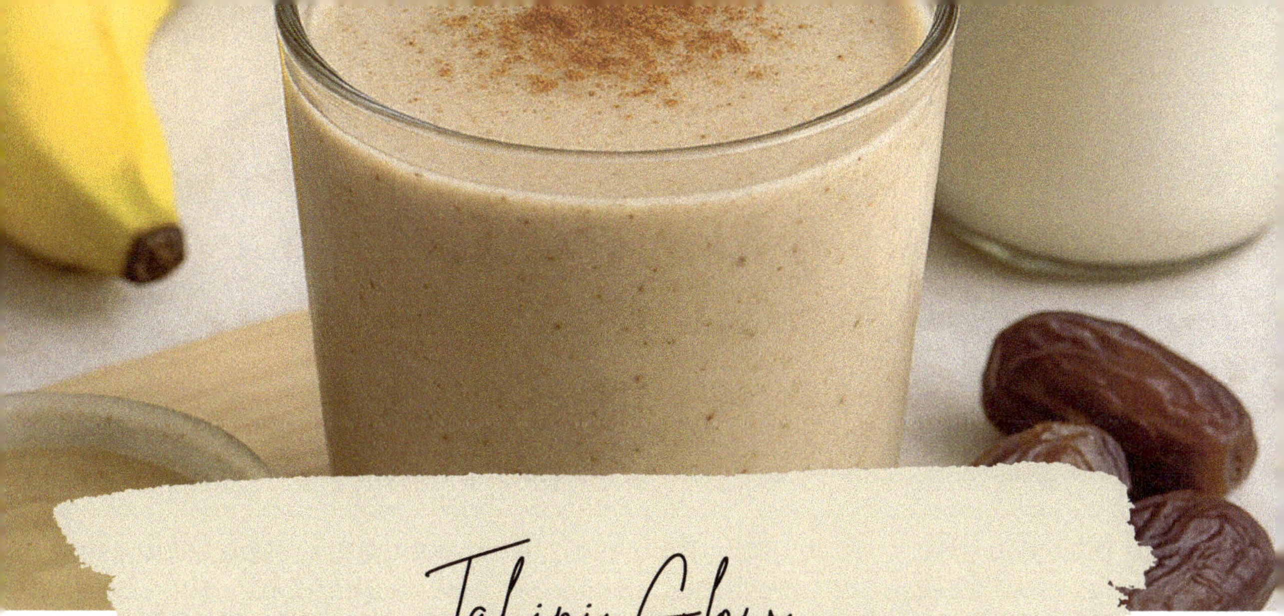

Tahini Glow

Tahini, banana, oat milk, dates, cinnamon

Tahini Glow Smoothie is a creamy and nutritious blend that combines the rich flavor of tahini with the sweetness of banana, the creaminess of oat milk, and the natural sweetness of dates. Enhanced with a hint of cinnamon, this smoothie is not only delicious but also packed with essential nutrients like calcium and magnesium, making it great for muscle and nerve repair.

INGREDIENTS:

- 2 tablespoons tahini
- 1 medium ripe banana
- 1 cup unsweetened oat
- 2-3 Medjool dates,
- 1/2 teaspoon ground cinnamon

OPTIONAL ADD-INS:

- 1 tablespoon chia seeds or flaxseeds: For added fiber and omega-3 fatty acids.
- 1/2 teaspoon vanilla extract: For extra flavor depth.
- Ice cubes: For a colder, refreshing smoothie.

INSTRUCTIONS:

1. If using whole dates, pit them and chop them into smaller pieces for more effortless blending. Peel the banana and break it into chunks for a smoother blending experience. Measure out the tahini, oat milk, cinnamon, and any optional ingredients as needed.

2. In a high-speed blender, combine the tahini, banana, unsweetened oat milk, chopped dates, and ground cinnamon. If you're using optional ingredients like chia seeds, flaxseeds, or ice cubes, add them now.

3. Blend on high until the mixture is entirely smooth and creamy, about 30-60 seconds. Ensure everything is well blended, stopping to scrape down the sides if needed. If the smoothie is too thick for your liking, add a little more oat milk to achieve your desired consistency. Taste your Tahini Glow Smoothie. If you prefer a sweeter taste, you can add more dates or honey (if you're not avoiding refined sugars) and blend again. Adjust the cinnamon based on your flavor preference for a stronger spice note.

4. Pour the smoothie into a glass or a to-go container. For a decorative touch, you can garnish with a sprinkle of cinnamon or a few chopped nuts on top. Enjoy immediately for the best flavor and nutritional benefits!

TIPS:

- This smoothie is perfect as a nutrient-dense breakfast option or an afternoon snack to keep you energized throughout the day.

- Feel free to experiment with adding other ingredients, such as spinach, for an extra boost of vitamins without significantly altering the flavor.

- You can prepare the ingredients in advance for a quick and easy smoothie preparation in the morning.

> *Enjoy your nourishing and flavorful Tahini Glow Smoothie, packed with essential nutrients for a healthy lifestyle!*

What does wellness mean to you today?

Day 18: Root & Rebuild

Believe in your power; you are worthy of all that you desire.

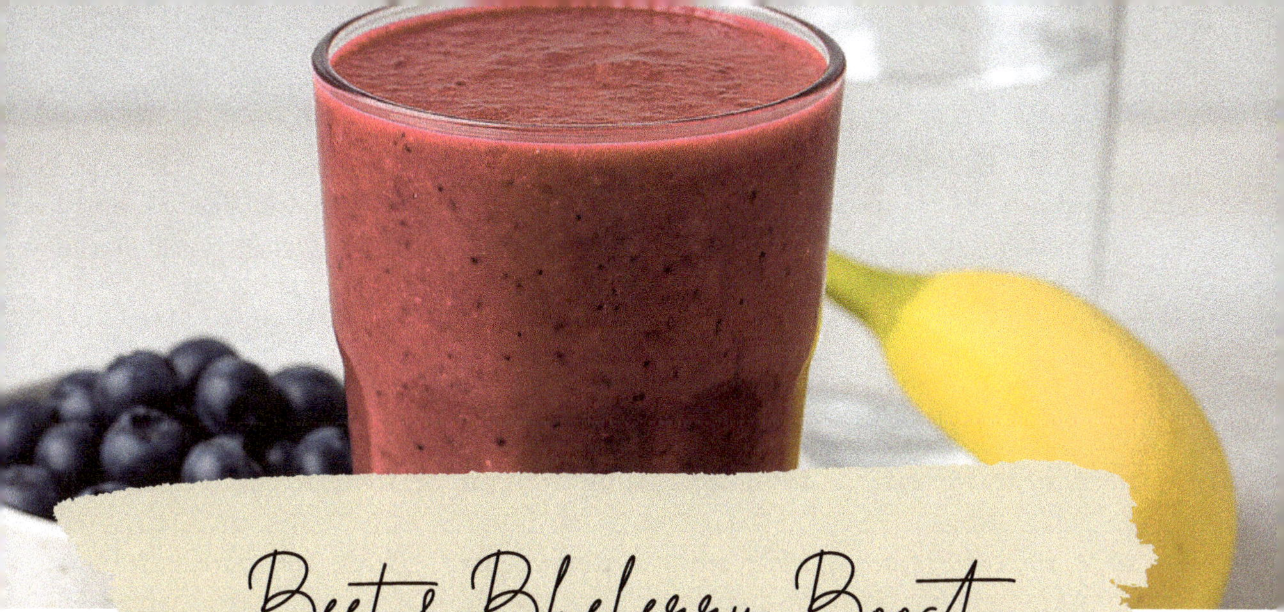

Beet & Blueberry Boost

Beet, blueberries, banana, chia, water

Beet & Blueberry Boost Smoothie is a vibrant and nutrient-dense drink that not only tastes delicious but also delivers a powerful combination of antioxidants and health benefits. With the earthy sweetness of beets, the tangy burst of blueberries, and the creaminess of bananas, this smoothie is perfect for improving circulation and providing a refreshing energy boost.

INGREDIENTS:

- 1 medium beet, peeled and chopped
- 1 cup fresh or frozen blueberries
- 1 medium ripe banana
- 2 tablespoons chia seeds
- 1 cup filtered water

OPTIONAL ADD-INS:

- 1 tablespoon honey or maple syrup: For added sweetness if desired.
- 1/2 teaspoon vanilla extract: For extra flavor depth. - A handful of spinach or kale: For added nutrients without significantly changing the flavor.
- Ice cubes: For a colder, refreshing smoothie.

INSTRUCTIONS:

1. Peel and chop the beet into small pieces (you can wear gloves to avoid staining your hands). Wash the blueberries thoroughly if you are using fresh ones. If using frozen, you can add them directly to the blender. Peel the banana and break it into chunks for more effortless blending. Measure out the chia seeds and water.

2. In a high-speed blender, add the chopped beet, blueberries, banana, chia seeds, and filtered water. If using any optional ingredients, such as honey, vanilla extract, or ice cubes, add those now as well. Blend on high until the mixture is completely smooth and creamy, which should take about 30-60 seconds. Stop and scrape down the sides if necessary to ensure all ingredients are well combined. If the smoothie is too thick, you can add a little more water to reach your desired consistency.

3. Taste your Beet & Blueberry Boost Smoothie. If you'd like it sweeter, consider adding more honey or maple syrup and blending again. Adjust the amount of beet or banana based on your taste preference. Pour the smoothie into a glass or a to-go container. For an optional garnish, you can sprinkle some extra chia seeds or a few blueberries on top. Enjoy immediately for the best flavor and maximum health benefits!

TIPS:

- This smoothie is perfect for a post-workout snack or as a nutritious breakfast option.
- You can prepare the ingredients ahead of time and store them in the refrigerator or freezer for a quick blend whenever needed.
- Experiment by adding other fruits or greens to customize the flavor and nutrient profile to your liking.

> *Enjoy your delightful and healthy.*
> *Beet & Blueberry Boost Smoothie!*

Day 18:
Root & Rebuild

I trust the pace of my becoming.

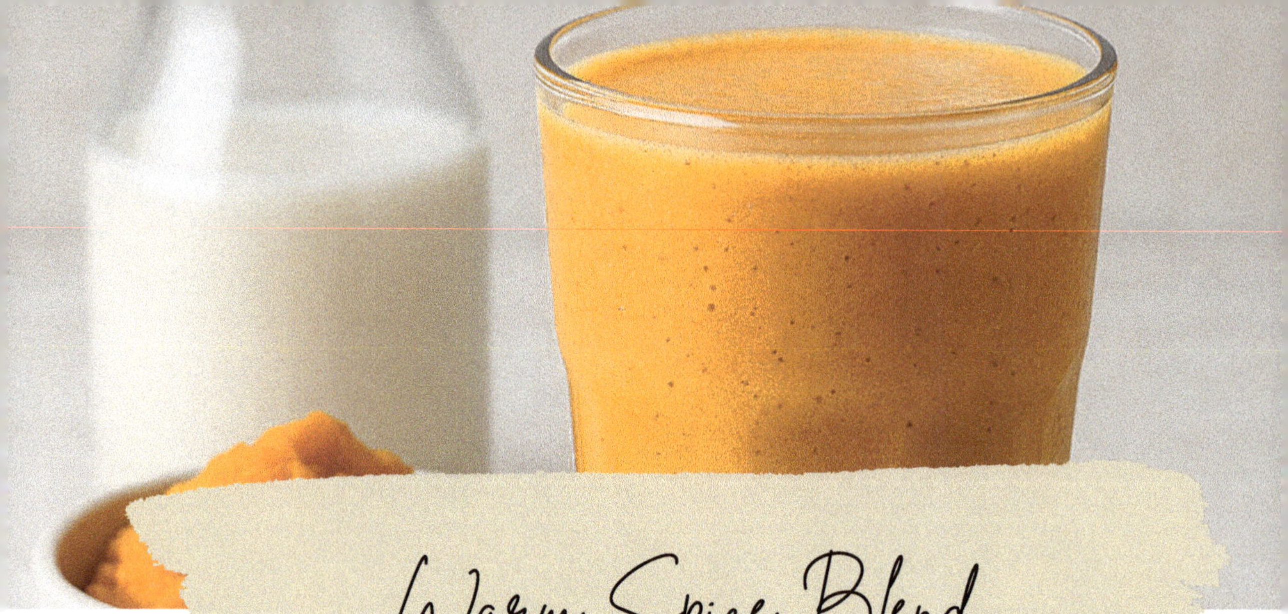

Warm Spice Blend

Pumpkin purée, almond milk, cinnamon, cardamom, vanilla

Warm Spice Blend Smoothie is a cozy and comforting drink that combines the rich flavors of pumpkin purée with warming spices like cinnamon and cardamom, along with creamy almond milk and a hint of vanilla. This delightful smoothie is perfect for chilly evenings or as a soothing treat at any time of year, and it's packed with fiber, making it both satisfying and nutritious.

INGREDIENTS:

- 1 cup pumpkin purée
- 1 cup unsweetened almond milk
- 1 teaspoon ground cinnamon
- 1/2 teaspoon ground cardamom
- 1/2 teaspoon vanilla extract

OPTIONAL ADD-INS:

- 1-2 tablespoons maple syrup or honey: For extra sweetness, if desired.
- 1 tablespoon chia seeds or flaxseeds: For added fiber and omega-3 fatty acids.
- A pinch of nutmeg: For an additional warm spice note.
- Ice cubes: For a chilled version.

INSTRUCTIONS:

1. Measure out the pumpkin purée, almond milk, spices, and any optional ingredients you wish to include. In a high-speed blender, add the pumpkin purée, unsweetened almond milk, ground cinnamon, ground cardamom, and vanilla extract. If you're using optional ingredients like sweetener, chia seeds, or ice cubes, incorporate them now. Blend on high speed until the ingredients are smooth and well combined, about 30 to 60 seconds. Scrape down the sides of the blender if necessary to ensure everything is thoroughly mixed.

2. Taste your Warm Spice Blend Smoothie. If you want it sweeter, add more maple syrup or honey and blend again. Add a pinch of nutmeg if you prefer a spicier flavor profile, and mix briefly to combine. Pour the smoothie into a glass or a cozy mug. If desired, you can garnish with a sprinkle of cinnamon or a light dusting of cardamom on top. Enjoy immediately for a comforting and nutritious treat!

TIPS:

- This smoothie is perfect for breakfast, a comforting afternoon snack, or a cozy treat before bed.

- You can make a larger batch and store it in the refrigerator for a quick grab-and-go option; just remember to give it a good shake before drinking.

- For added variety, feel free to experiment with other spices, such as ginger or cloves.

> *Enjoy your warm and nourishing Warm Spice Blend Smoothie, filled with comforting flavors and health benefits!*

What does wellness mean to you today?

Day 19: Restore *Your Fire*

Let gratitude guide your thoughts and transform your experiences

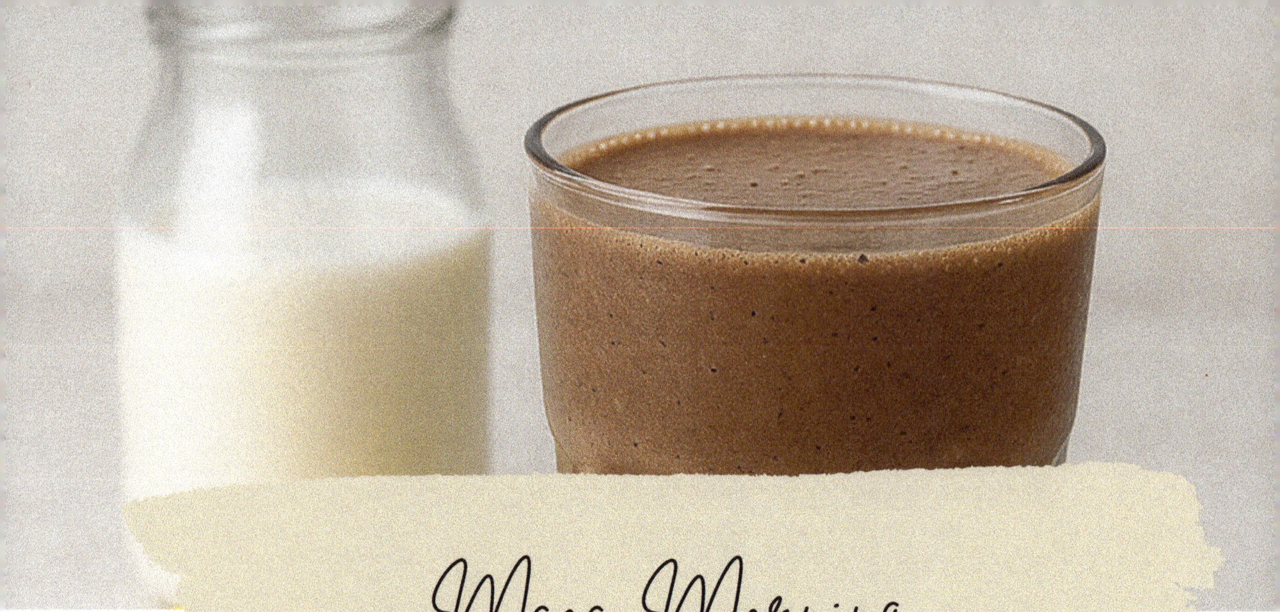

Maca Morning

Maca powder, banana, almond milk, cacao, flax

Maca Morning Smoothie is a delicious and energizing blend designed to kickstart your day. Combining the nutty flavor of maca powder with the sweetness of banana, the richness of cacao, and the smoothness of almond milk, this smoothie is not only flavorful but also packed with nutrients that help balance hormones and provide sustained energy. Flaxseeds give an extra boost of fiber and omega-3 fatty acids for a powerful morning start.

INGREDIENTS:

- 2 teaspoons maca powder
- 1 medium ripe banana
- 1 cup unsweetened almond milk
- 1 tablespoon unsweetened cacao powder
- 1 tablespoon ground flaxseeds

OPTIONAL ADD-INS:

- 1 tablespoon honey or maple syrup: For added sweetness if desired.
- 1/2 teaspoon vanilla extract: For extra flavor depth.
- A handful of spinach: For added nutrients without significantly altering the flavor.
- Ice cubes: For a chilled, refreshing smoothie.

INSTRUCTIONS:

1. Peel the banana and break it into chunks for more effortless blending. Measure out the maca powder, cacao powder, ground flaxseeds, and almond milk. In a high-speed blender, add the banana, maca powder, cacao powder, almond milk, and ground flaxseeds. If you're using any optional ingredients, such as honey, vanilla extract, or ice cubes, add them now. Blend on high until everything is smooth and creamy, about 30-60 seconds. Make sure to scrape down the sides if needed to ensure all ingredients are well combined. If the smoothie is too thick for your liking, you can add a little more almond milk to reach your desired consistency.

2. Taste your Maca Morning Smoothie. If you'd like it sweeter, you can add more honey or maple syrup and blend again. Adjust the cacao and maca powder according to your taste preference. Pour the smoothie into a glass or a to-go container. For a decorative touch, you can sprinkle a little extra cacao powder or flaxseed on top. Enjoy immediately to benefit from the fresh ingredients and their nutrients!

TIPS:

- This smoothie is perfect for breakfast or as a mid-morning snack to energize your day.
- Feel free to customize the smoothie by adding other fruits or leafy greens based on your preference.
- You can prepare ingredients in advance for a quick smoothie on busy mornings.

> *Enjoy your energizing and hormone-balancing Maca Morning Smoothie!*

Day 19:
Restore *Your Fire*

Stillness is where my strength grows.

Coconut Lavender Ease

Coconut milk, lavender, pineapple, banana

The Coconut Lavender Ease Smoothie is a delightful, cooling drink that combines the creamy texture of coconut milk with the floral notes of lavender, the tropical sweetness of pineapple, and the smoothness of banana. This soothing smoothie is perfect for a refreshing treat, promoting relaxation and emotional well-being.

INGREDIENTS:

- 1 cup coconut milk
- 1 teaspoon dried culinary lavender
- 1 cup fresh or frozen pineapple chunks
- 1 medium ripe banana

OPTIONAL ADD-INS:

- 1 tablespoon honey or maple syrup: For added sweetness if desired.
- 1/2 teaspoon vanilla extract: To enhance flavor.
- A handful of spinach: For added nutrients without altering the taste.
- Ice cubes: For a colder, refreshing smoothie.

INSTRUCTIONS:

1. If using fresh pineapple, chop it into chunks. If using frozen pineapple, there is no need to thaw it. Peel the banana and break it into chunks for more effortless blending. Measure out the coconut milk and lavender. Infuse the Lavender (Optional) If you want a stronger lavender flavor, you can infuse the coconut milk by heating it gently on the stove or in the microwave until warm (but not boiling), and then steep the dried lavender in it for about 10-15 minutes. Strain out the lavender before using it.

2. In a high-speed blender, add the coconut milk (infused or not), pineapple chunks, banana, and dried lavender. If you're using any optional ingredients, like honey, vanilla extract, or ice cubes, add them now. Blend on high until the mixture is completely smooth and creamy, about 30 to 60 seconds. Stop and scrape down the sides if necessary to ensure all ingredients are well combined. If the smoothie is too thick, you can add a small amount of coconut milk or cold water to achieve your desired consistency.

3. Taste your Coconut Lavender Ease Smoothie. If you'd like it sweeter, you can add more honey or maple syrup and blend again. Adjust the amount of lavender according to your taste preference. Pour the smoothie into a glass or a to-go container. For a decorative touch, you can garnish with a sprinkle of lavender or a slice of pineapple on the rim. Enjoy immediately to experience the full benefits and flavors!

TIPS:

- This smoothie is perfect for a refreshing snack on a hot day or as part of a calming nighttime routine.
- Feel free to experiment with other fruits, such as mango or berries, to create a distinct flavor profile.
- Preparing the ingredients ahead of time can make for a quick and easy smoothie whenever you need a refreshing treat.

> *Enjoy your Coconut Lavender Ease Smoothie, designed to cool and soothe both your body and mind!*

What does wellness mean to you today?

Day 20:
Digest & Declutter

Prioritize self-care and watch your spirit soar.

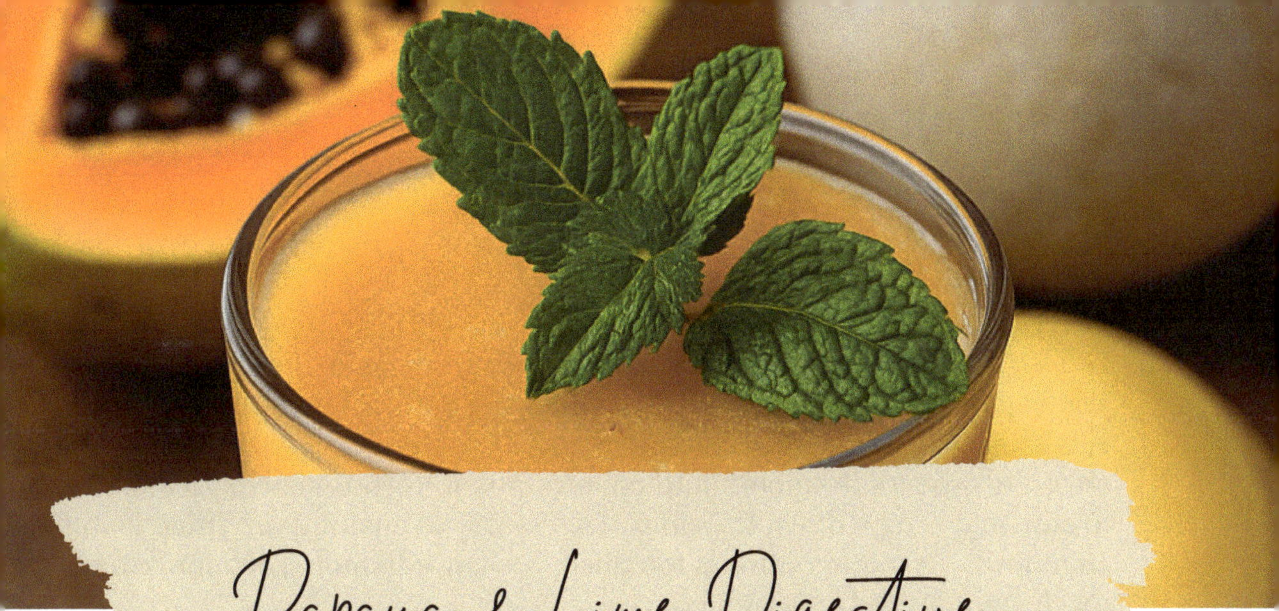

Papaya & Lime Digestive

Papaya, lime, mint, ginger, coconut water

The Papaya & Lime Digestive Smoothie is a refreshing and zesty blend designed to support digestion and provide relief from bloating. With the digestive enzymes from papaya, the tanginess of lime, the freshness of mint, and a kick of ginger, this smoothie is perfect for starting your day with a bit of extra pep and a healthy boost.

INGREDIENTS:

- 1 cup ripe papaya, peeled and diced
- Juice of 1 lime
- A handful of fresh mint leaves
- 1-inch piece of fresh ginger, peeled and grated
- 1 cup coconut water

OPTIONAL ADD-INS:

- 1 tablespoon chia seeds or flaxseeds: For additional fiber and omega-3 fatty acids.
- 1 tablespoon honey or agave syrup: For a sweeter taste.
- Ice cubes: For a colder and more refreshing smoothie.

INSTRUCTIONS:

1. Peel and dice the papaya, removing the seeds. Squeeze the juice from the lime, discarding any seeds. Rinse the mint leaves and pat them dry. - Peel and grate the ginger.

2. In a high-speed blender, add the diced papaya, lime juice, fresh mint leaves, grated ginger, and coconut water. If using any optional ingredients, such as chia seeds, honey, or ice cubes, add them to the blender now. Blend on high until the mixture is smooth and creamy, about 30-60 seconds. Make sure to stop and scrape down the sides if necessary to ensure everything is well combined. - If the smoothie is too thick, you can add more coconut water to reach your desired consistency.

3. Taste your Papaya & Lime Digestive Smoothie. If you'd like it sweeter, you can add more honey or agave and blend again. Adjust the amount of lime and ginger to suit your flavor preference. Pour the smoothie into a glass or a to-go container. Garnish with a sprig of fresh mint or a lime wedge if desired.

4. Enjoy immediately for the best flavor and health benefits!

TIPS:

- This smoothie is perfect for breakfast or as a refreshing drink whenever you need digestive support.

- Experiment with adding other digestive-friendly ingredients, such as spinach or kale, for added nutritional benefits without compromising flavor.

- You can prepare the ingredients ahead of time for a quick and easy morning smoothie.

> *Enjoy your delightful and digestive-friendly Papaya & Lime Digestive Smoothie!*

Day 20: Digest & Declutter

My wellness is not a luxury—it is my birthright.

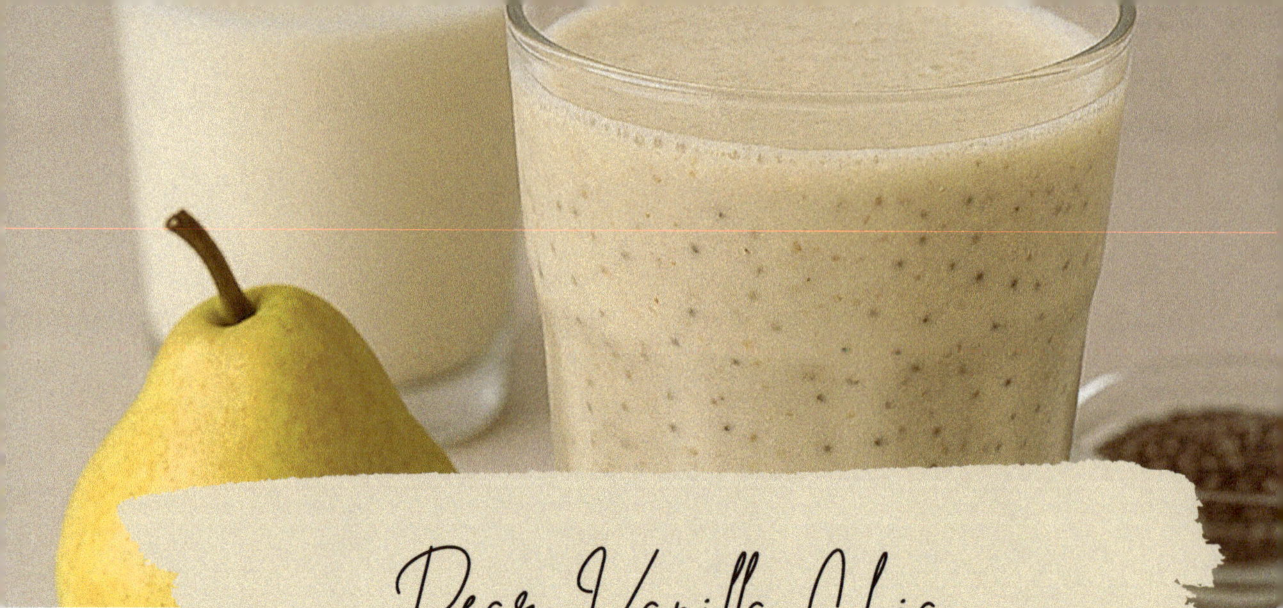

Pear Vanilla Chia

Pear, almond milk, vanilla, chia

The Pear Vanilla Chia Smoothie is a delicious and nutritious drink designed to support gut health and promote gentle elimination. Combining the natural sweetness of pear with the creamy texture of almond milk, a hint of vanilla, and the fiber-rich benefits of chia seeds, this smoothie is not only satisfying but also beneficial for digestive wellness.

INGREDIENTS:

- 1 ripe pear, cored and
- 1 cup unsweetened almond
- 1/2 teaspoon vanilla extract
- 2 tablespoons chia seeds

OPTIONAL ADD-INS:

- 1 tablespoon honey or maple syrup: For extra sweetness, if desired.
- 1/2 banana: For added creaminess and natural sweetness.
- A pinch of cinnamon: For flavor and additional digestive benefits.
- Ice cubes: If you prefer a colder smoothie.

INSTRUCTIONS:

1. Wash and chop the pear, removing the core. You can leave the skin on for additional fiber. Measure out the almond milk, vanilla extract, and chia seeds. In a high-speed blender, add the chopped pear, almond milk, chia seeds, and vanilla extract. If you're using any optional ingredients, like honey, banana, cinnamon, or ice cubes, add them now. Blend on high until the mixture is smooth and creamy, which should take about 30-60 seconds. Ensure that you scrape down the sides if necessary to ensure all ingredients are well combined. - If the smoothie is too thick, you can add more almond milk to achieve your desired consistency.

2. Taste your Pear Vanilla Chia Smoothie. If you'd like it sweeter, add more honey or maple syrup and blend again. Adjust the amount of vanilla or cinnamon according to your flavor preference. Pour the smoothie into a glass or a to-go container. For an optional garnish, you can sprinkle a few chia seeds on top. Enjoy immediately to benefit from its fresh flavors and gut-friendly properties!

3. Enjoy immediately for the best flavor and health benefits!

TIPS:

- This smoothie is an excellent breakfast option or a light snack that supports digestive health

- You can prepare the ingredients ahead of time and store them in the refrigerator to make blending quick and easy.

- Experiment with adding other fruits or leafy greens to enhance nutrition without significantly altering the flavor.

> *Enjoy your nutritious and gut-friendly Pear Vanilla Chia Smoothie!*

What does wellness mean to you today?

Day 21: Rest & Reflect

Dare to dream big and take bold steps toward your vision.

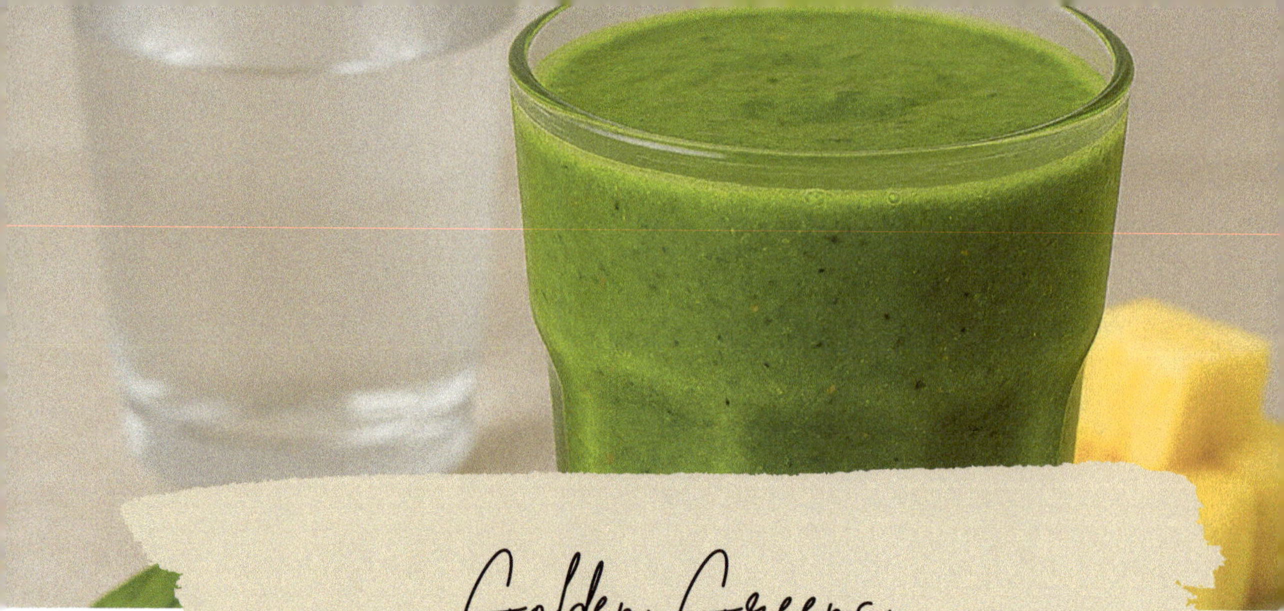

Golden Greens

Spinach, pineapple, turmeric, lemon, coconut water

The Golden Greens Smoothie is a vibrant and nutrient-rich drink designed to energize and refresh you while providing a wealth of health benefits. Combining the sweetness of pineapple with the earthy richness of spinach, the anti-inflammatory properties of turmeric, and a zing of lemon, this smoothie is not only delicious but also packed with antioxidants and electrolytes.

INGREDIENTS:

- 2 cups fresh spinach leaves
- 1 cup fresh or frozen pineapple chunks
- 1 teaspoon ground turmeric
- Juice of 1 lemon
- I cup of coconut water

OPTIONAL ADD-INS:

- 1 tablespoon chia seeds or flaxseeds: For added fiber and omega-3 fatty acids.
- 1 tablespoon honey or maple syrup: For an additional touch of sweetness.
- A handful of mint leaves for a refreshing aroma and flavor.
- Ice cubes: If you prefer a chilled smoothie.

INSTRUCTIONS:

1. Rinse the spinach leaves thoroughly and remove any tough stems. If using fresh pineapple, peel, core, and chop it into chunks. If using frozen pineapple, you can add it directly to the blender. Cut the lemon in half and squeeze out the juice, discarding any seeds. Measure out the ground turmeric and coconut water.

2. In a high-speed blender, add thc spinach, pineapple chunks, ground turmeric, lemon juice, and coconut water. If using optional ingredients like chia seeds, honey, mint leaves, or ice cubes, add those as well. Blend on high until the mixture is completely smooth and creamy, about 30 to 60 seconds. Stop and scrape down the sides of the blender as needed to ensure everything is well combined. If the smoothie is too thick for your liking, add more coconut water to achieve your desired consistency.

3. Taste your Golden Greens Smoothie. If you prefer a sweeter taste, feel free to add more honey or maple syrup and blend again. Adjust the amount of turmeric or lemon juice based on your flavor preferences. Pour the smoothie into a glass or a to-go container. For an additional garnish, you can sprinkle a little extra turmeric on top or add a slice of lemon. Enjoy immediately to maximize flavor and nutritional benefits!

TIPS:

- This smoothie is perfect for a refreshing breakfast, an energizing snack, or a post-workout recovery drink.

- You can prepare the ingredients ahead of time for a quick and easy blend in the morning.

- Experiment with adding other fruits or leafy greens to customize the flavor and nutritional profile to your liking.

> *Enjoy your invigorating and nourishing Golden Greens Smoothie, bursting with flavor and a wealth of health benefits!*

“

Day 21: Rest & Reflect

*Even when I pause,
I am still progressing.*

”

Evening Restore

Warm oat milk, chamomile tea, date, cinnamon

The Evening Restore Smoothie is a calming and soothing drink designed to help you wind down and prepare for a restful night's sleep. Combining warm oat milk with chamomile tea, a naturally sweet date, and a sprinkle of cinnamon, this cozy blend is ideal for promoting relaxation and enhancing a sense of well-being.

INGREDIENTS:

- 1 cup warm oat milk (avoid boiling)
- 1/2 cup brewed chamomile tea (cooled to warm)
- 1 Medjool date,
- 1/2 teaspoon ground

OPTIONAL ADD-INS:

- A pinch of nutmeg: For an additional warm spice note that promotes relaxation.
- 1/4 teaspoon vanilla extract: For extra flavor depth.
- 1 tablespoon chia seeds or flaxseeds: To boost fiber and omega-3 fatty acids for added nutritional benefits.
- Ice cubes: If you prefer a chilled version (though warm is recommended for bedtime).

INSTRUCTIONS:

1. Brew chamomile tea using a tea bag or loose chamomile flowers. Let it steep for about 5-7 minutes. After brewing, strain out the flowers if necessary and let them cool slightly. In a small saucepan, gently warm the oat milk over low heat until it's warm but not boiling. Alternatively, you can microwave it for about 30-60 seconds.

2. In a high-speed blender, add the warm oat milk, brewed chamomile tea (cooled to warm), pitted date, and ground cinnamon. If you're using optional ingredients like nutmeg, vanilla extract, or chia seeds, add them now. Blend on high until the mixture is smooth and creamy, about 30 to 45 seconds. Ensure that the date is thoroughly blended into the mixture. If you prefer a thicker texture, you can add a few ice cubes and blend again until smooth.

3. Taste your Evening Restore Smoothie. If you'd like it sweeter, feel free to add another date or a drizzle of honey and blend again. Adjust the spices to your preference if desired. Pour the smoothie into a cozy mug or a glass. For a decorative touch, consider sprinkling a little extra cinnamon or nutmeg on top. Enjoy your smoothie warm as part of your bedtime relaxation ritual.

TIPS:

- This smoothie is perfect for winding down after a long day and can be a satisfying conclusion to your evening routine.

- Prepare the chamomile tea and other ingredients ahead of time to make blending quick and easy right before bed.

- Feel free to experiment with additional herbs or spices, such as lavender or cardamom, for a unique twist.

> *Enjoy your calming and restorative Evening Restore Smoothie before a peaceful night's sleep!*

What does wellness mean to you today?

Restore & *Hydrate Check-In*

> *Healing, balance, softness, self-trust*

I am a Divine Original

In what ways did I allow softness, grace, and healing into my life this week? Where have I witnessed growth in the stillness?

Day 22: Glow *From Within*

Let go of what no longer serves you; make space for love and joy.

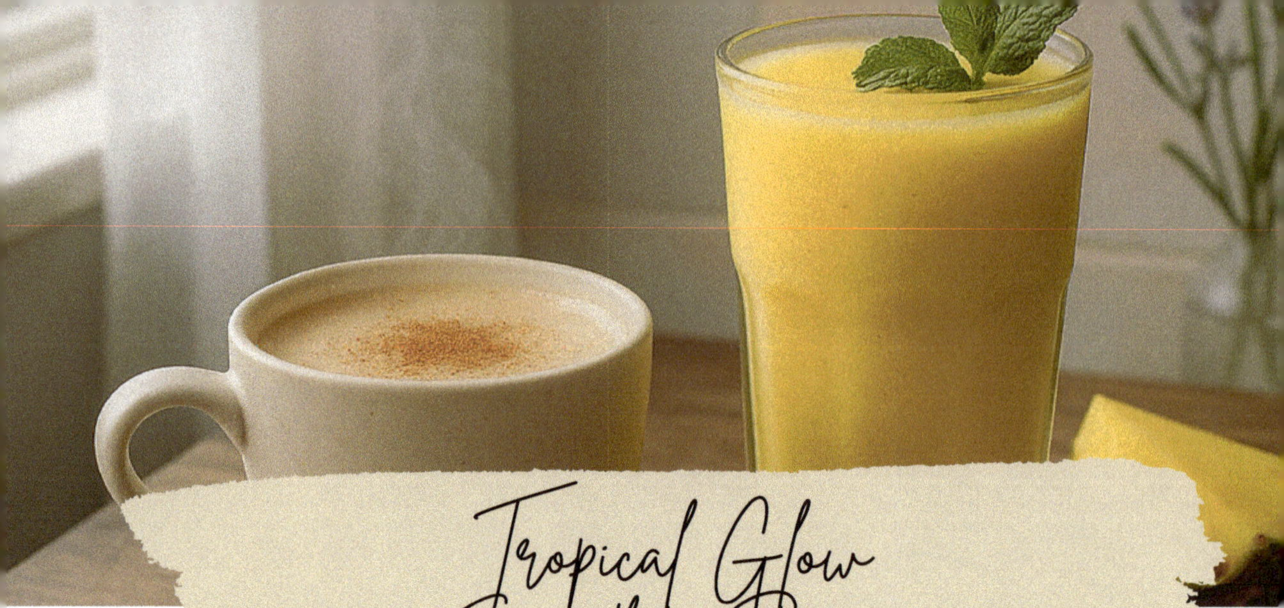

Tropical Glow Smoothie Recipe

Pineapple, mango, lime, coconut water, mint

The Tropical Glow Smoothie is a vibrant and refreshing blend packed with the delicious flavors of pineapple, mango, lime, and coconut water, along with a touch of fresh mint. This smoothie is perfect for brightening your skin and providing deep hydration, making it an excellent choice for a refreshing breakfast or midday snack.

INGREDIENTS:

- 1 cup fresh pineapple chunks
- 1 ripe mango, peeled and diced
- Juice of 1 lime
- 1 cup coconut water
- A handful of fresh mint leaves

OPTIONAL ADD-INS:

- 1 tablespoon chia seeds or flaxseeds: For additional fiber and omega-3 fatty acids.
- 1 tablespoon honey or agave syrup: For added sweetness.
- Ice cubes: For an extra-chilled smoothie.

INSTRUCTIONS:

1. Peel and chop the mango into small pieces. If using fresh pineapple, peel and chop it into chunks. Wash the mint leaves and pat them dry. Cut the lime in half and squeeze out the juice, discarding any seeds. In a high-speed blender, add the pineapple chunks, diced mango, lime juice, coconut water, and fresh mint leaves. If using optional ingredients like chia seeds, honey, or ice cubes, add them now. Blend on high until the mixture is completely smooth and creamy, about 30-60 seconds. Make sure to stop and scrape down the sides if necessary to ensure everything is well combined. If the smoothie is too thick for your liking, you can add a little more coconut water to achieve your desired consistency.

2. Taste your Tropical Glow Smoothie. If you'd like it sweeter, feel free to add more honey or agave syrup and blend briefly. Adjust the mint based on your preference for a stronger mint flavor if desired. Pour the smoothie into a glass or a to-go container. Garnish with a sprig of fresh mint or a slice of lime on the rim if desired. Enjoy immediately for the best flavor and hydration benefits!

TIPS:

- This smoothie is perfect as a refreshing breakfast option, a midday pick-me-up, or a delicious post-workout drink.

- Feel free to customize the recipe by adding other tropical fruits, such as banana or passion fruit, for added flavor.

- Preparing and chopping ingredients in advance can make for a quicker and easier smoothie-making experience.

> *Enjoy your vibrant and hydrating Tropical Glow Smoothie for a delicious boost to your day!*

Day 22:
Glow *From Within*

I don't chase the glow—I create it.

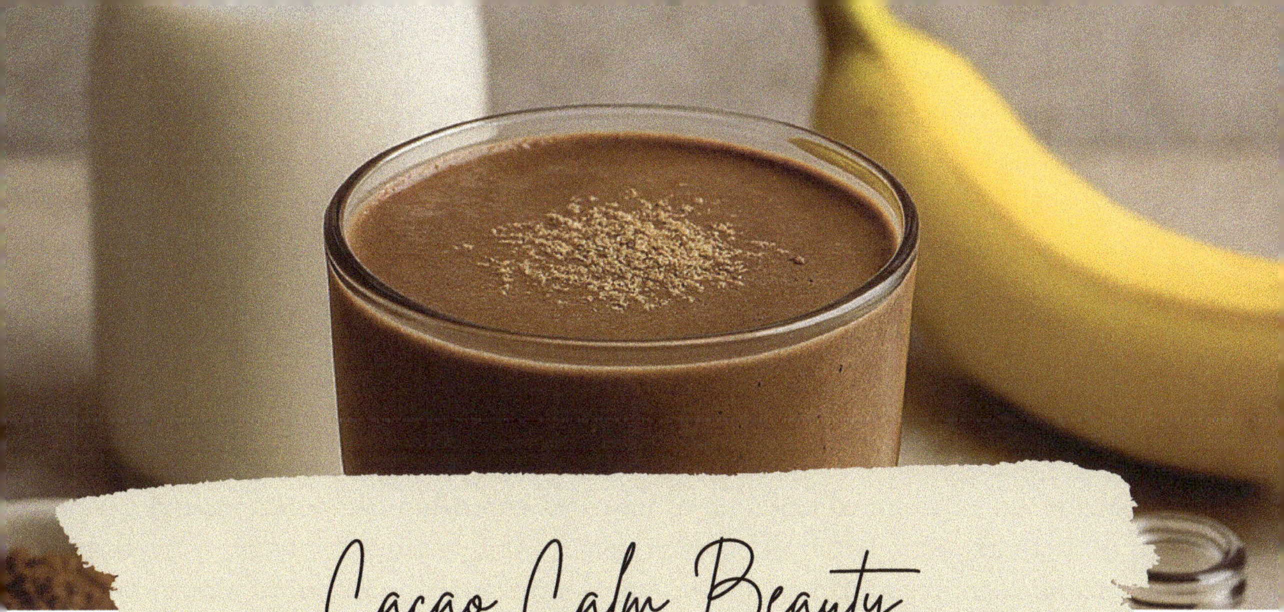

Cacao Calm Beauty

Cacao powder, almond milk, banana, flax, vanilla

The Cacao Calm Beauty Smoothie is a rich and delightful drink that combines the luscious flavor of cacao with the creaminess of almond milk, the natural sweetness of banana, and the nutritional benefits of flaxseed. This smoothie is not only delicious but also mood-boosting and supportive of healthy hormonal balance, making it an ideal choice for a beauty-enhancing breakfast or snack.

INGREDIENTS:

- 2 tablespoons cacao powder
- 1 cup unsweetened almond milk
- 1 medium ripe banana
- 1 tablespoon ground flaxseed
- 1/2 teaspoon vanilla extract

OPTIONAL ADD-INS:

- 1 tablespoon honey or maple syrup: For additional sweetness, if desired.
- A sprinkle of cinnamon For warmth and extra flavor.
- A handful of spinach: For added nutrients without altering the flavor.
- Ice cubes: For a chilled smoothie.

INSTRUCTIONS:

1. Peel the banana and break it into chunks for more effortless blending. Measure out the cacao powder, almond milk, ground flaxseed, and vanilla extract.

2. In a high-speed blender, add the almond milk, cacao powder, banana chunks, ground flaxseed, and vanilla extract. If you're using any optional ingredients, such as honey, cinnamon, spinach, or ice cubes, add them now. Blend on high speed until the mixture is smooth and creamy, about 30 to 60 seconds. Stop to scrape down the sides if necessary to ensure everything is well combined. If the smoothie is too thick, add a bit more almond milk to reach your desired consistency.

3. Taste your Cacao Calm Beauty Smoothie. If you prefer a sweeter taste, feel free to add more honey or maple syrup and blend again. - Adjust the cacao to your taste preference for a richer chocolate flavor, if desired. Pour the smoothie into a glass or a to-go container. For an optional garnish, you can sprinkle a little extra cacao powder or flaxseed on top.

TIPS:

- This smoothie is perfect for a nutritious breakfast or as an afternoon snack to keep your energy levels stable.
- You can customize the smoothie by adding other fruits or protein sources based on your dietary preferences.
- Preparing the ingredients ahead of time can streamline your morning routine and make smoothie preparation quick and easy.

> *Enjoy your delicious and hormone-supporting Cacao Calm Beauty Smoothie!*

What does wellness mean to you today?

Day 23: Radiant *Strength*

Shhhh....Listen to your body; it knows what you need to thrive.

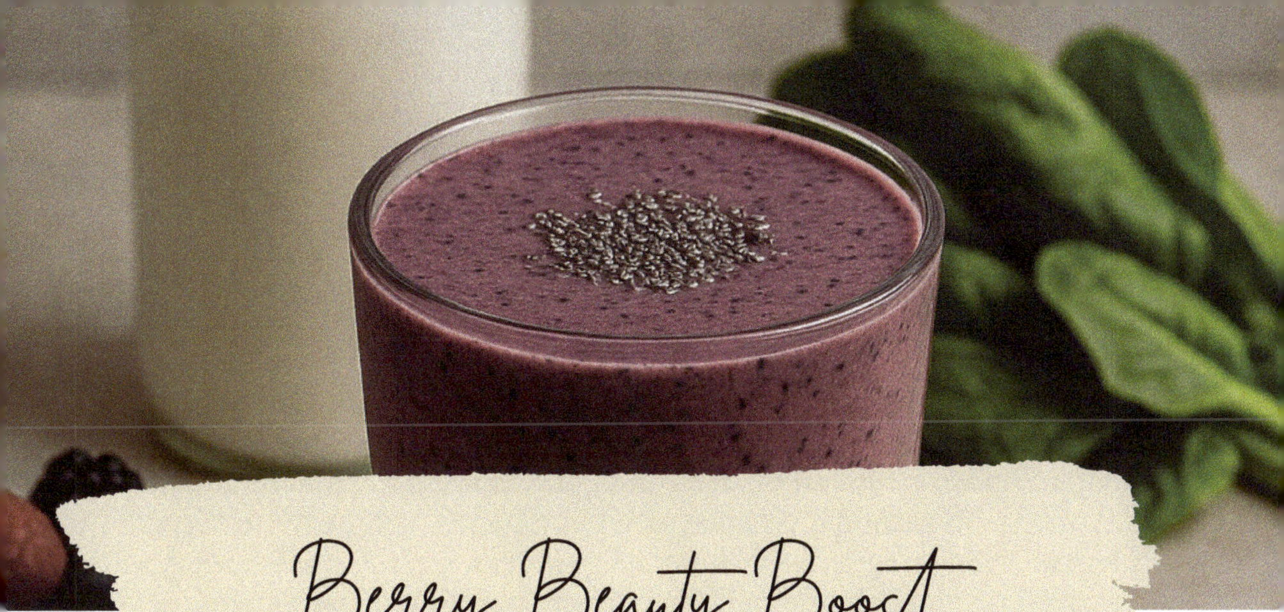

Berry Beauty Boost

Mixed berries, chia seeds, spinach, almond milk

The Berry Beauty Boost Smoothie is a vibrant and nutrient-dense drink that combines mixed berries, chia seeds, spinach, and almond milk. This delicious smoothie is not only packed with antioxidants to support skin health but also rich in fiber for digestive wellness. It's perfect for a nutritious breakfast or a post-workout snack.

INGREDIENTS:

- 1 cup mixed berries (fresh or frozen)
- 2 tablespoons chia seeds
- 1 cup fresh spinach
- 1 cup unsweetened almond milk

OPTIONAL ADD-INS:

- 1 tablespoon honey or maple syrup: For added sweetness, if desired.
- 1/2 banana: For extra creaminess and natural sweetness.
- 1/2 teaspoon vanilla extract: For added depth of flavor.
- Ice cubes: If you prefer a colder, thicker smoothie.

INSTRUCTIONS:

1. Wash the mixed berries thoroughly if using fresh berries. If using frozen, they can be added directly to the blender. Rinse the spinach leaves and pat them dry. Measure out the almond milk, chia seeds, and any optional ingredients as needed.

2. In a high-speed blender, add the mixed berries, chia seeds, spinach, and almond milk. If using optional ingredients like honey, banana, or ice cubes, add them now. Blend on high until the mixture is smooth and creamy, about 30-60 seconds. You may need to stop and scrape down the sides to ensure everything is well combined. If the smoothie is too thick, you can add a little more almond milk to achieve your desired consistency.

3. Taste your Berry Beauty Boost Smoothie. If you'd like it sweeter, consider adding more honey or maple syrup and blending again. Adjust the amount of spinach to achieve a different nutrient profile without significantly altering the flavor. Pour the smoothie into a glass or a to-go container. For a decorative touch, you can garnish with a few whole berries or a sprinkle of chia seeds on top.

TIPS:

- This smoothie is great for meal prep; consider making a larger batch to enjoy throughout the week.

- You can add protein powder for an extra protein boost, especially if you're using it as a post-workout recovery drink.

- Consider blending in other greens, such as kale or Swiss chard, for added nutritional variety.

> *Enjoy your delicious and nutrient-packed Berry Beauty Boost Smoothie, perfect for nourishing your body and skin!*

Day 23: Radiant *Strength*

This light you see?
I built it from within.

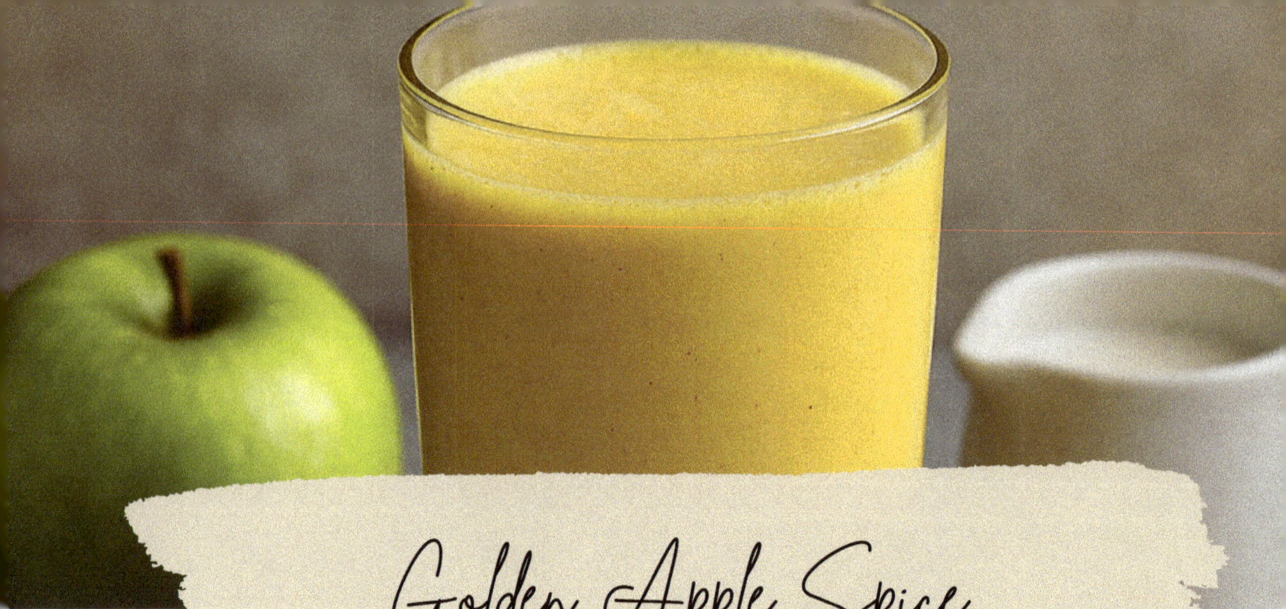

Golden Apple Spice

Green apple, ginger, turmeric, cinnamon, oat milk

The Golden Apple Spice Smoothie is a vibrant and nourishing drink that combines the crispness of green apple with the warm, earthy flavors of ginger and turmeric, complemented by the sweetness of cinnamon and the creaminess of oat milk. This smoothie is perfect for those looking to support gut health and combat inflammation, making it an excellent choice for breakfast or as a refreshing snack.

INGREDIENTS:

- 1 medium green apple, cored and chopped
- 1-inch piece of fresh ginger, peeled and grated
- 1 teaspoon ground turmeric
- 1/2 teaspoon ground cinnamon
- 1 cup unsweetened oat milk

OPTIONAL ADD-INS:

- 1 tablespoon honey or maple syrup: If you prefer additional sweetness.
- 1 tablespoon chia seeds or flaxseeds: For added fiber and omega-3 fatty acids.
- A pinch of black pepper: To enhance the absorption of turmeric's beneficial compounds.
- Ice cubes: If you prefer a colder, refreshing smoothie.

INSTRUCTIONS:

1. Wash the green apple and chop it into chunks, leaving the skin on for additional fiber. Peel and grate the ginger. Measure out the turmeric, cinnamon, and oat milk.

2. In a high-speed blender, add the chopped green apple, grated ginger, ground turmeric, ground cinnamon, and oat milk. If using any optional ingredients, such as honey, chia seeds, black pepper, or ice cubes, add them now. Blend on high until the mixture is smooth and creamy, about 30-60 seconds. Stop to scrape down the sides if necessary to ensure everything is well combined. If the smoothie is too thick for your liking, you can add a little more oat milk to achieve your desired consistency.

3. Taste your Golden Apple Spice Smoothie. If you'd like it sweeter, feel free to add more honey or maple syrup and blend again. Adjust the amount of ginger or cinnamon based on your flavor preference. Pour the smoothie into a glass or a to-go container. For a decorative touch, you can garnish with a sprinkle of cinnamon or a slice of apple.

4. Enjoy immediately for the best flavor and health benefits!

TIPS:

- This smoothie is ideal for starting your day on a healthy note or as a refreshing afternoon pick-me-up.

- You can prepare the ingredients in advance for quick assembly in the morning.

- Feel free to experiment with other fruits or greens to customize the flavor profile to your liking.

Enjoy your delicious and health-boosting Golden Apple Spice Smoothie!

What does wellness mean to you today?

Day 24: Step *Into Shine*

Every day is a new opportunity to align with your purpose.

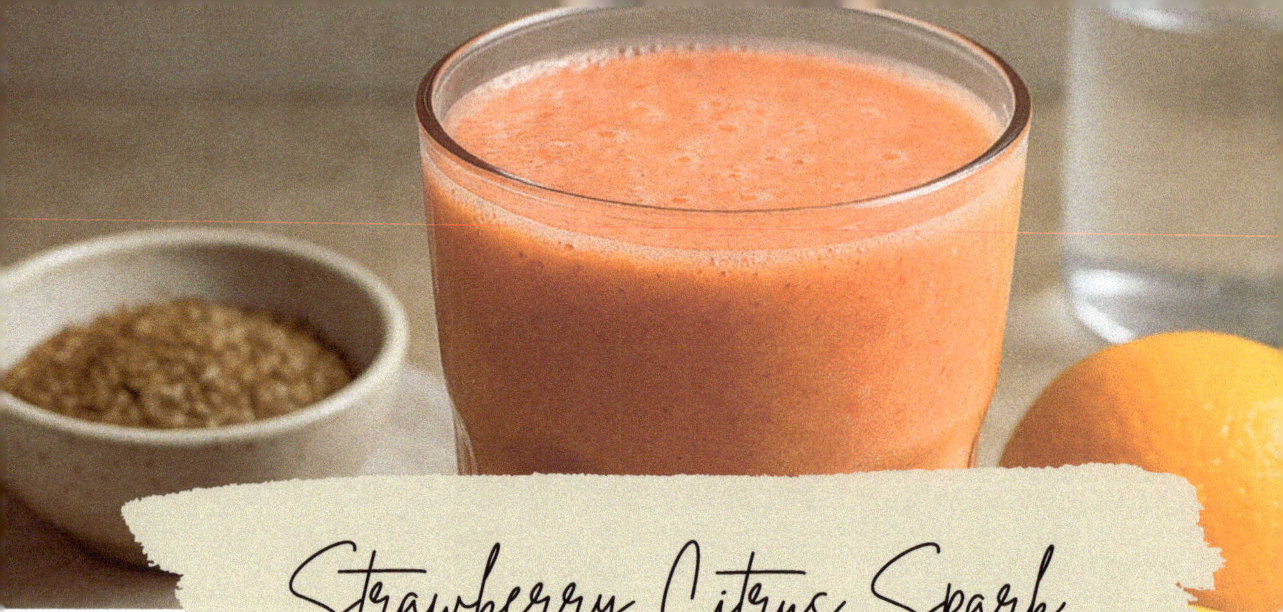

Strawberry Citrus Spark

Strawberries, orange, lemon, flaxseed, water

The Strawberry Citrus Spark Smoothie is a refreshing and vibrant blend that combines the sweetness of strawberries with the zesty brightness of orange and lemon. This delightful smoothie is loaded with vitamin C, making it perfect for supporting skin health and boosting your immune system. Flaxseeds add a crunchy texture while providing fiber and omega-3 fatty acids.

INGREDIENTS:

- 1 cup fresh strawberries, hulled and chopped
- 1 medium orange, peeled and segmented
- Juice of 1 lemon
- 2 tablespoons ground flaxseed
- 1 cup filtered water

OPTIONAL ADD-INS:

- 1 tablespoon honey or maple syrup: For additional sweetness, if desired.
- 1/2 banana: For extra creaminess and natural sweetness.
- Ice cubes: For a chilled smoothie.

INSTRUCTIONS:

1. Wash the strawberries and hull them. Chop them into smaller pieces for more effortless blending. Peel and segment the orange, removing any seeds. Cut the lemon in half and squeeze out the juice, discarding any seeds.

2. In a high-speed blender, add the chopped strawberries, orange segments, lemon juice, ground flaxseed, and filtered water. If you're using optional ingredients, such as honey, banana, or ice cubes, add them now. Blend on high speed until the mixture is completely smooth and creamy, about 30 to 60 seconds. Stop and scrape down the sides if necessary to ensure that all ingredients are well-mixed. If the smoothie is too thick, you can add more water to reach your desired consistency.

3. Taste your Strawberry Citrus Spark Smoothie. If you'd like it sweeter, feel free to add more honey or maple syrup and blend again. Adjust the citrus flavors by adding more lemon juice if you prefer a more tart taste. Pour the smoothie into a glass or a to-go container. For a decorative touch, you can garnish with a slice of orange or a few whole strawberries.

TIPS:

- This smoothie is perfect for a refreshing breakfast or a nutritious snack to energize your day. You can experiment with other fruits or greens based on your taste preferences and nutritional needs. Preparing your ingredients in advance can save time in the morning and make smoothie-making quicker and easier.

> *Enjoy the refreshing and nourishing Strawberry Citrus Spark Smoothie!*

Day 24:
Step *Into Shine*

*Joy is my natural state—
I am reclaiming it.*

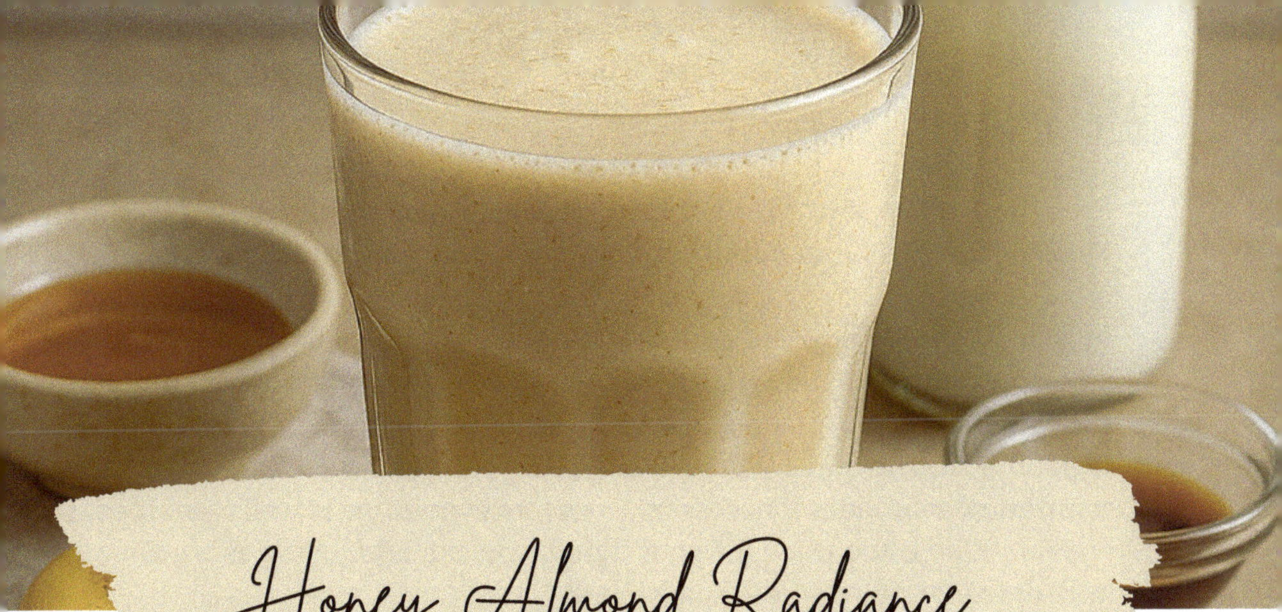

Honey Almond Radiance

Almond milk, banana, honey, cinnamon, vanilla

The Honey Almond Radiance Smoothie is a deliciously creamy and nourishing drink that combines almond milk, banana, honey, cinnamon, and vanilla to create a sweet treat that supports balanced blood sugar levels and promotes healthy skin. This smoothie is perfect for breakfast or as a refreshing snack anytime during the day.

INGREDIENTS:

- 1 cup unsweetened almond milk
- 1 medium ripe banana
- 1-2 tablespoons honey
- 1/2 teaspoon ground cinnamon
- 1/2 teaspoon vanilla extract

OPTIONAL ADD-INS:

- 1 tablespoon chia seeds or flaxseeds: For added fiber and omega-3 fatty acids.
- 1 tablespoon almond butter: For added protein and creaminess.
- A pinch of sea salt: To enhance flavor.
- Ice cubes: If you prefer a colder, refreshing smoothie.

INSTRUCTIONS:

1. Peel the banana and break it into chunks for more effortless blending. Measure out the almond milk, honey, cinnamon, and vanilla extract.

2. In a high-speed blender, add the almond milk, banana chunks, honey, ground cinnamon, and vanilla extract. If using any optional ingredients, such as chia seeds, almond butter, or ice cubes, add them now. Blend on high until smooth and creamy, about 30-60 seconds. Make sure to stop and scrape down the sides if necessary to ensure everything is well combined. If the smoothie is too thick for your liking, you can add a little more almond milk to reach your desired consistency.

3. Taste your Honey Almond Radiance Smoothie. If you'd like it sweeter, feel free to add more honey and blend again. Adjust the cinnamon based on your preference for a spicier flavor. Pour the smoothie into a glass or a to-go container. For a decorative touch, you can sprinkle a little extra cinnamon on top or garnish with a banana slice.

TIPS:

- This smoothie is perfect for a nutritious breakfast or a quick snack that helps maintain energy throughout the day.

- Feel free to customize the smoothie by adding other ingredients, such as spinach or protein powder, to increase its nutrient density.

- Prepare the ingredients in advance for a quick blend on busy mornings.

Enjoy your nourishing and delicious. Honey Almond Radiance Smoothie!

What does wellness mean to you today?

Day 25: Celebrate You!

Being true to yourself is the ultimate expression of freedom.

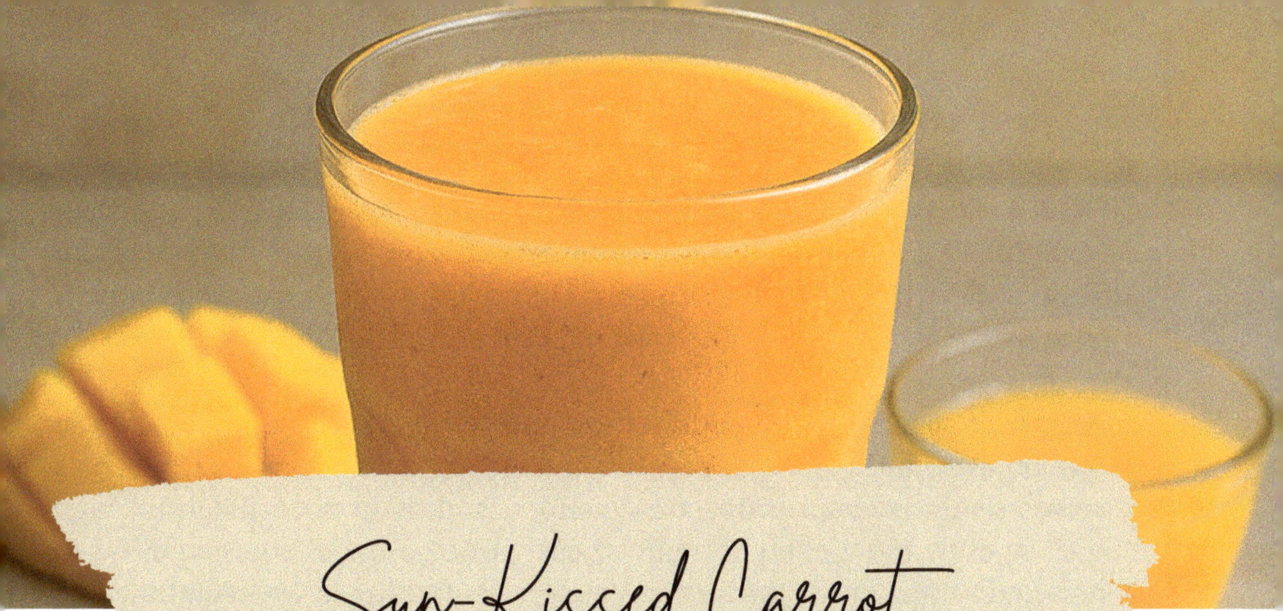

Sun-Kissed Carrot

Carrot, mango, orange juice, ginger

The Sun-Kissed Carrot Smoothie is a vibrant and delicious blend designed to brighten your skin and support gut health. Combining the natural sweetness of carrots and mango with zesty orange juice and a hint of ginger, this smoothie is packed with nutrients and antioxidants. It's perfect for a refreshing breakfast or a rejuvenating snack any time of day.

INGREDIENTS:

- 1 medium carrot, peeled and chopped
- 1 cup ripe mango, peeled and diced
- 1/2 cup fresh orange juice
- 1-inch piece of fresh ginger, peeled and grated

OPTIONAL ADD-INS:

- 1 tablespoon honey or maple syrup: For added sweetness, if desired.
- 1 tablespoon chia seeds or flaxseeds: For extra fiber and omega-3 fatty acids.
- 1/2 cup coconut water or almond milk: For added hydration and creaminess, if you prefer a smoother texture.
- Ice cubes: If you prefer a colder, refreshing smoothie.

INSTRUCTIONS:

1. Wash and peel the carrot, then chop it into smaller pieces for more effortless blending. Peel and dice the mango, removing the pit. Squeeze the juice from fresh oranges if using whole oranges. Otherwise, you can use store-bought juice (preferably without added sugar). Peel and grate the ginger.

2. In a high-speed blender, add the chopped carrot, diced mango, fresh orange juice, and grated ginger. If using any optional ingredients, such as honey, seeds, coconut water, or ice cubes, add them now. Blend on high until smooth and creamy, usually about 30-60 seconds. You may need to stop and scrape down the sides to ensure everything is well combined. If the smoothie is too thick, you can add more orange juice or a liquid of your choice (such as coconut water or almond milk) to achieve your desired consistency.

3. Taste your Sun-Kissed Carrot Smoothie. If you'd like it sweeter, you can add more honey or maple syrup and blend again. Adjust the amount of ginger according to your preference for a spicier taste. Pour the smoothie into a glass or a to-go container. For added flair, consider garnishing with a slice of mango or carrot on the rim.

TIPS:

- This smoothie is an excellent choice for a nutritious breakfast or a midday snack that keeps you energized and supports digestion.

- You can prepare your ingredients ahead of time and store them in the fridge or freezer for a quick and easy smoothie whenever you need it.

- Experiment with adding other fruits or greens to customize the flavor and nutrition of the smoothie!

> *Enjoy your refreshing and vibrant Sun-Kissed Carrot Smoothie!*

Day 25: Celebrate *You!*

My presence is powerful, even in quiet moments.

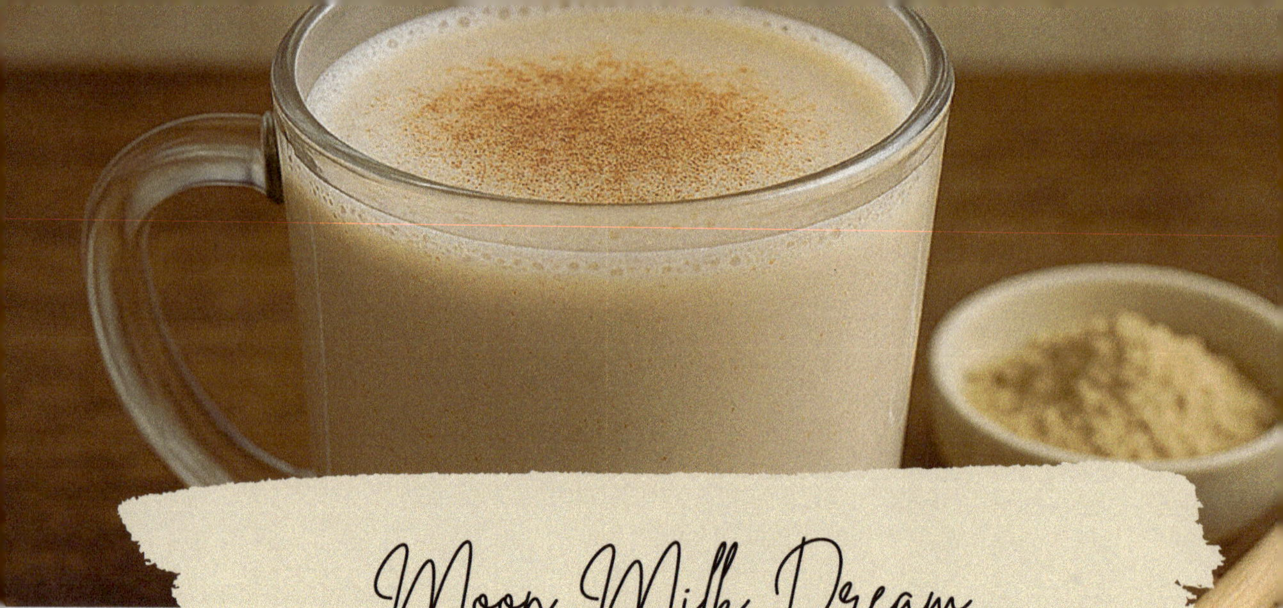

Moon Milk Dream

Warm oat milk, ashwagandha, cinnamon, honey

The Moon Milk Dream Smoothie is a warm, soothing beverage designed to help you relax and unwind while providing emotional clarity and support. Combining warm oat milk with the adaptogenic properties of ashwagandha, the warmth of cinnamon, and a touch of honey for sweetness, this smoothie makes for a delightful bedtime treat that promotes restful sleep and reduces stress.

INGREDIENTS:

- 1 cup warm oat milk
- 1 teaspoon ashwagandha powder
- 1/2 teaspoon ground
- 1-2 tablespoons honey

OPTIONAL ADD-INS:

- A pinch of nutmeg: For additional warmth and flavor depth.
- - 1/4 teaspoon vanilla extract: To enhance flavor.
- 1 tablespoon chia seeds: For added fiber and omega-3 fatty acids (optional, note that chia seeds will thicken the drink).

INSTRUCTIONS:

1. In a small saucepan, gently heat the oat milk over low heat until warm but not boiling. You can also heat it in the microwave for about 30-60 seconds.

2. In a blender, combine the warm oat milk, ashwagandha powder, ground cinnamon, and honey. If you're using optional ingredients like nutmeg, vanilla extract, or chia seeds, add them now. Blend on low to medium speed just until combined, about 15 to 30 seconds. If using chia seeds, blend for a little longer to help incorporate them into the mixture.

3. Taste your Moon Milk Dream Smoothie. If you prefer a sweeter taste, you can add more honey and blend briefly to incorporate it. Pour the smoothie into a cozy mug. For a decorative touch, you can sprinkle a little cinnamon or nutmeg on top. Enjoy warm baths as part of your evening routine to promote relaxation and a sense of calm.

TIPS:

- This smoothie is perfect for calming your mind and preparing for sleep, making it a great addition to your nighttime routine.

- Feel free to experiment with flavors by adding other spices, such as cardamom, for a unique taste profile.

- You can prepare the oat milk and other ingredients in advance to make blending quick and easy before bed.

> *Enjoy your soothing and restorative Moon Milk Dream Smoothie for a peaceful night's sleep!*

What does wellness mean to you today?

Day 26:
Own *Your Glow*

Live fully, love deeply, and recognize the beauty in every moment.

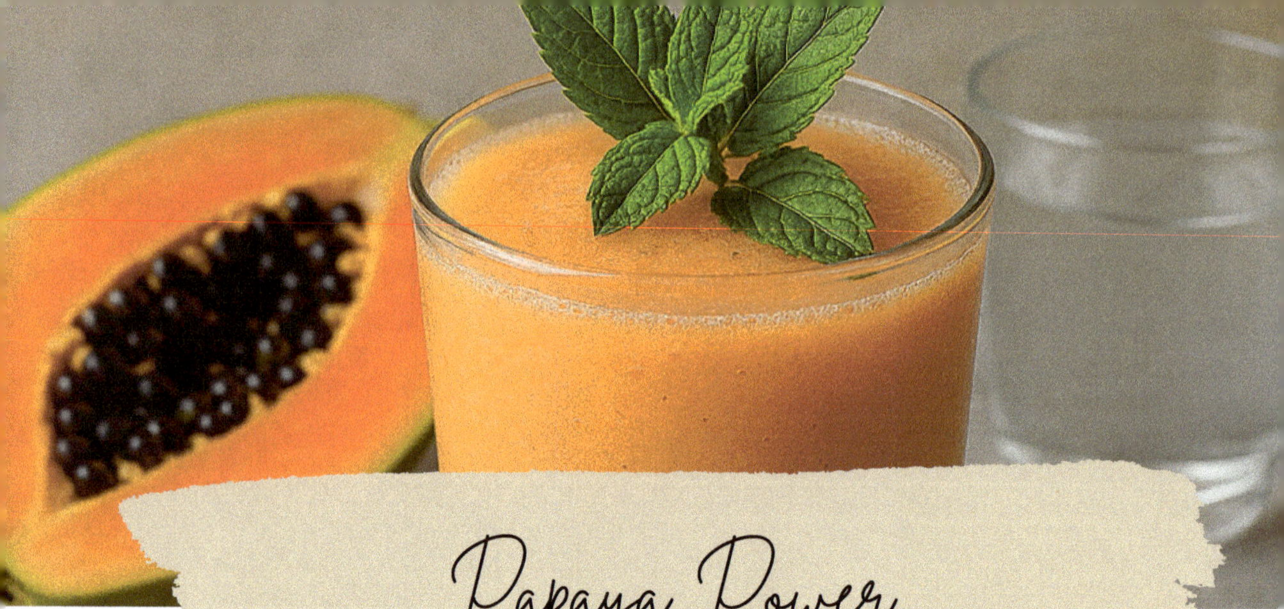

Papaya Power

Papaya, lime, mint, coconut water

The Papaya Power Smoothie is a refreshing and nutrient-packed drink that combines the tropical flavors of papaya, lime, and mint with hydrating coconut water. This smoothie is rich in digestive enzymes and antioxidants, making it excellent for promoting digestive health and reducing inflammation. It's perfect for breakfast or as a revitalizing snack during the day.

INGREDIENTS:

- 1 cup ripe papaya, peeled and diced
- Juice of 1 lime
- A handful of fresh mint leaves
- 1 cup coconut water

OPTIONAL ADD-INS:

- 1 tablespoon chia seeds or flaxseeds: For added fiber and omega-3 fatty acids.
- 1 tablespoon honey or agave syrup: For those who prefer extra sweetness.
- Ice cubes: For a colder, refreshing smoothie.

INSTRUCTIONS:

1. Peel and dice the ripe papaya, removing the seeds. Juice the lime and set it aside. Wash the fresh mint leaves thoroughly.

2. In a high-speed blender, add the diced papaya, lime juice, fresh mint leaves, and coconut water. If using any optional ingredients, such as chia seeds, honey, or ice cubes, add them now. Blend on high until the mixture is smooth and creamy, about 30-60 seconds. Scrape down the sides of the blender as needed to ensure everything is well combined. If the smoothie is too thick for your liking, you can add more coconut water to achieve your desired consistency.

3. Taste your Papaya Power Smoothie. If you'd like it sweeter, feel free to add more honey or agave syrup and blend briefly. Pour the smoothie into a glass or to-go container. You can garnish with a sprig of mint or a slice of lime for a decorative touch.

TIPS:

- This smoothie is fantastic as a refreshing breakfast or as a post-workout recovery drink.

- You can prepare the ingredients in advance for a quick and easy smoothie assembly in the morning.

- Feel free to experiment with other tropical fruits, such as bananas or mangoes, for added flavors and nutrients.

> *Enjoy your refreshing and digestive-friendly Papaya Power Smoothie!*

"

Day 26: Own *Your Glow*

*When I feel good,
I shine without apology.*

"

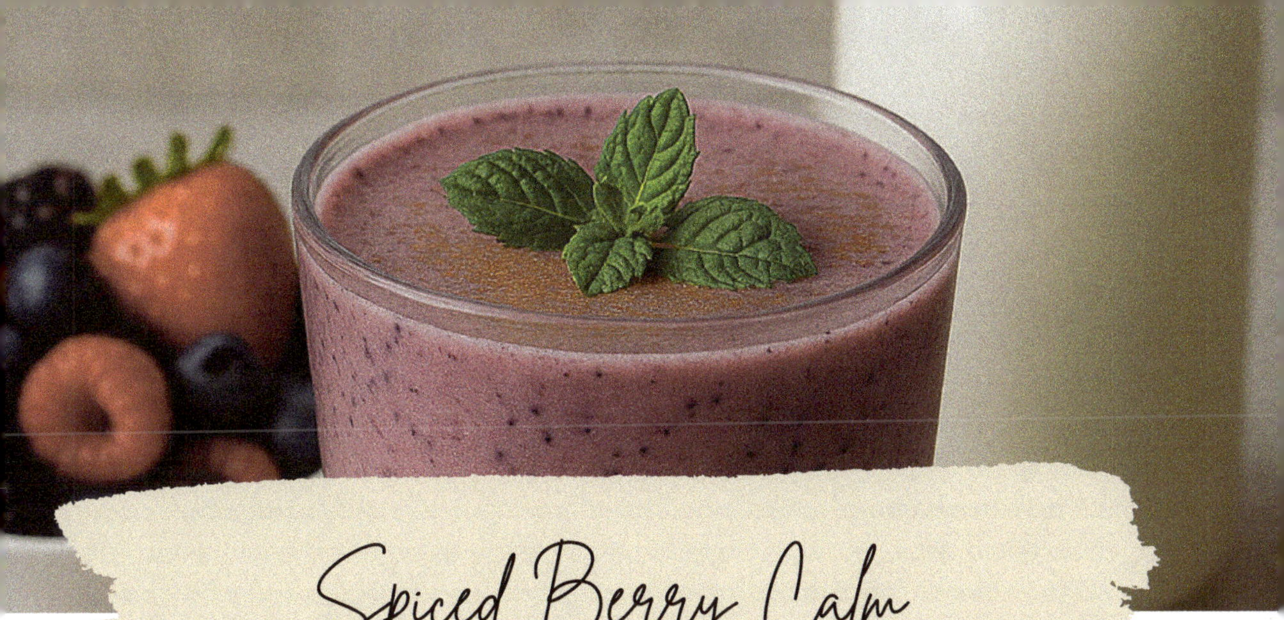

Spiced Berry Calm

Mixed berries, almond milk, cinnamon, nutmeg

The Spiced Berry Calm Smoothie is a delicious blend that combines the sweetness of mixed berries with the creamy goodness of almond milk, enhanced by warm spices like cinnamon and nutmeg. This smoothie is not only refreshing but also packed with antioxidants, making it an excellent option for promoting healthy skin and stabilizing energy levels throughout the day.

INGREDIENTS:

- 1 cup mixed berries (fresh or frozen)
- 1 cup unsweetened almond milk
- 1/2 teaspoon ground cinnamon
- 1/4 teaspoon ground nutmeg

OPTIONAL ADD-INS:

- 1 tablespoon honey or maple syrup: For added sweetness, if desired.
- 1 tablespoon chia seeds or flaxseeds: For added fiber and omega-3 fatty acids.
- A handful of spinach: For extra nutrients without altering the flavor.
- Ice cubes : If you prefer a colder smoothie.

INSTRUCTIONS:

1. If using fresh berries, wash them thoroughly to remove any dirt or debris. If using frozen berries, you can add them directly to the blender. Measure out the almond milk, cinnamon, and nutmeg.

2. In a high-speed blender, add the mixed berries, almond milk, ground cinnamon, and ground nutmeg. If you're using any optional ingredients, such as honey, chia seeds, or ice cubes, add them now. Blend on high until the mixture is completely smooth and creamy, about 30 to 60 seconds. Stop to scrape down the sides if necessary to ensure everything is well combined. - If the smoothie is too thick, you can add a little more almond milk to reach your desired consistency.

3. Taste your Spiced Berry Calm Smoothie. If you'd like it sweeter, consider adding more honey or maple syrup and blend again. Adjust the spices according to your preference for a stronger taste. Pour the smoothie into a glass or a to-go container. For an optional garnish, consider sprinkling a little extra cinnamon or nutmeg on top.

TIPS:

- This smoothie is perfect for breakfast or a midday snack that will keep you energized and satisfied.

- Feel free to customize the recipe by adding other favorite fruits or greens.

- Preparing the ingredients in advance can streamline your morning routine and make it easier to blend your smoothie quickly.

> *Enjoy your nourishing and anti-aging Spiced Berry Calm Smoothie!*

What does wellness mean to you today?

Day 27: Radiate *Ease*

Your unique journey is your greatest gift; embrace it wholeheartedly

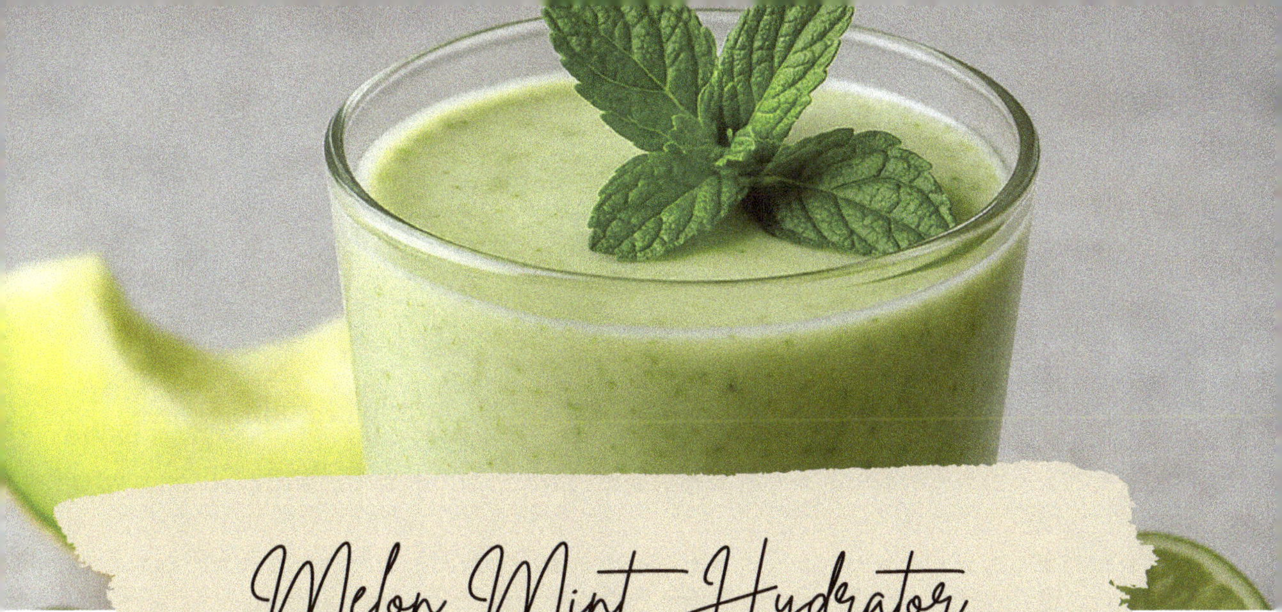

Melon Mint Hydrator

Honeydew or cantaloupe, mint, cucumber, lime

The Melon Mint Hydrator Smoothie is a refreshing and hydrating drink that combines the sweet flavors of honeydew or cantaloupe with cooling cucumber, zesty lime, and fragrant mint. This delightful smoothie is perfect for quenching your thirst and revitalizing your skin, making it an excellent choice for hot days or post-workout refreshments.

INGREDIENTS:

- 1 cup honeydew or cantaloupe, diced
- 1/2 cucumber, peeled and chopped
- Juice of 1 lime
- A handful of fresh mint leaves

OPTIONAL ADD-INS:

- 1 tablespoon honey or agave syrup: For additional sweetness, if desired.
- 1 tablespoon chia seeds: For added fiber and omega-3 fatty acids.
- Ice cubes: For a chilled smoothie.

INSTRUCTIONS:

1. If using honeydew or cantaloupe, peel and seed the melon, then dice it into cubes. Peel and chop the cucumber into smaller pieces. Squeeze the juice from the lime, discarding any seeds. Wash the mint leaves and pat them dry.

2. In a high-speed blender, combine the diced melon, chopped cucumber, lime juice, and fresh mint leaves. If you're using any optional ingredients, such as honey or chia seeds, add them now. Blend on high until the mixture is smooth and creamy, about 30-60 seconds. Scrape down the sides if necessary to ensure everything is well-mixed. If the smoothie is too thick, you can add a little more water or coconut water to achieve your desired consistency.

3. Taste your Melon Mint Hydrator Smoothie. If you'd like it sweeter, you can add more honey or agave syrup and blend again. Adjust the mint flavor to your liking by adding more mint leaves and mixing again. Pour the smoothie into a glass or a to-go container. For an extra touch, garnish with a sprig of fresh mint or a slice of lime on the rim. Enjoy immediately for the best flavor and hydration benefits!

TIPS:

- This smoothie is perfect for a refreshing breakfast, post-workout recovery, or a hydrating snack throughout the day.

- Feel free to experiment with other herbs, like basil, for a different flavor twist.

- Preparing ingredients in advance makes for a quick and easy smoothie on busy days.

> *Enjoy your refreshing and hydrating Melon Mint Hydrator Smoothie for a boost of freshness and vitality!*

Day 27: Radiate *Ease*

I am not shrinking—I am shining.

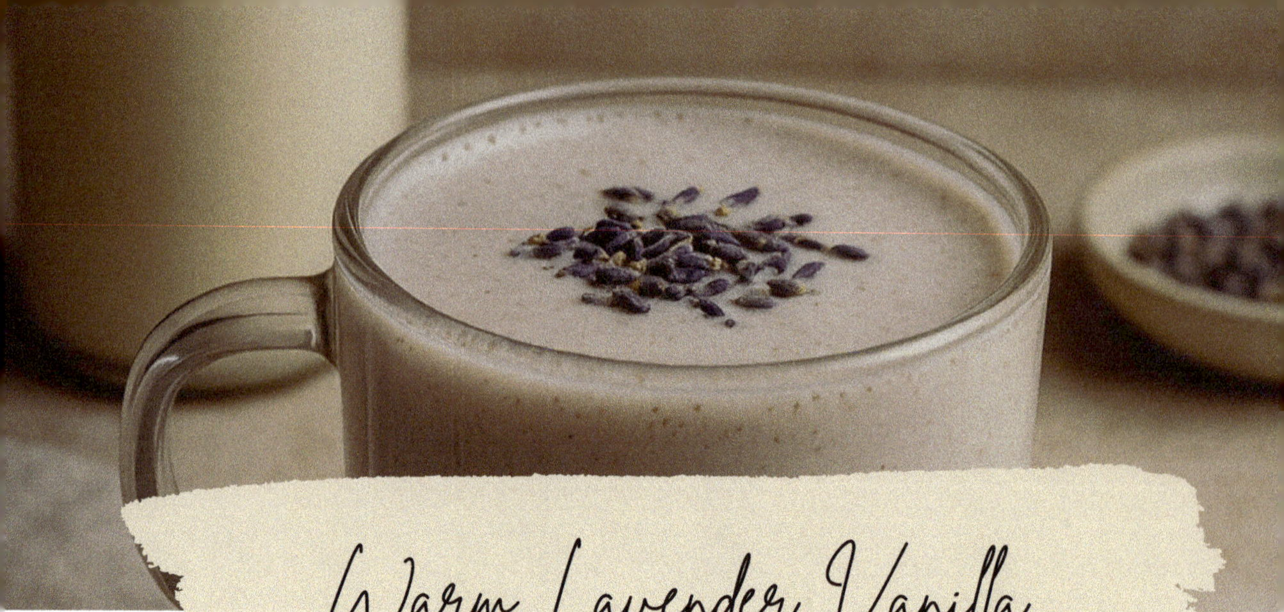

Warm Lavender Vanilla

Warm almond milk, vanilla, lavender, date

The Warm Lavender Vanilla Smoothie is a soothing drink perfect for winding down in the evening or as a comforting treat before bed. With the creamy texture of warm almond milk, the sweet notes of vanilla, and the calming properties of lavender, this smoothie promotes relaxation and a sense of tranquility. The addition of a date offers natural sweetness, making it a delightful bedtime beverage.

INGREDIENTS:

- 1 cup warm almond milk
- 1/2 teaspoon dried culinary lavender
- 1 Medjool date, pitted
- 1/2 teaspoon vanilla extract

OPTIONAL ADD-INS:

- A pinch of sea salt: To elevate the flavors and balance sweetness.
- 1/4 teaspoon ground cinnamon: For added warmth and flavor.
- 1 tablespoon chia seeds: For added fiber and omega-3 fatty acids.
- Ice cubes: If you want a chilled version, however, this smoothie is best enjoyed warm.

INSTRUCTIONS:

1. If you prefer a stronger lavender flavor, you can infuse the almond milk by heating it gently on the stove or in the microwave and steeping the dried lavender for about 10-15 minutes. Strain out the lavender before using it. In a small saucepan, gently warm the almond milk over low heat until it's warm but not boiling. Alternatively, you can heat it in the microwave for about 30-60 seconds.

2. In a high-speed blender, combine the warm almond milk, pitted dates, vanilla extract, and lavender (if you haven't infused the milk). If you're using any optional ingredients, such as a pinch of sea salt, cinnamon, or chia seeds, add them now. Blend on low to medium speed until the mixture is smooth and creamy, about 30 to 45 seconds. Ensure the date is completely blended into the mixture. If using chia seeds, blend a bit longer to incorporate them well.

3. Taste your Warm Lavender Vanilla Smoothie. If you'd like it sweeter, consider adding more date or a drizzle of honey and blend again. Adjust the flavor by adding a bit more vanilla or cinnamon if desired. Pour the smoothie into a cozy mug or a glass. For a decorative touch, you can garnish with a sprinkle of cinnamon or a few lavender buds on top. Enjoy warm as part of your bedtime routine for relaxation and comfort.

TIPS:

- This smoothie is perfect for winding down after a busy day and can be a lovely addition to your nighttime routine.

- You can adjust the consistency by adding more warm almond milk if you prefer a thinner smoothie.

- Feel free to experiment with other spices, such as nutmeg or adaptogen powders, for added benefits.

Enjoy your comforting and relaxing Warm Lavender Vanilla Smoothie!

What does wellness mean to you today?

Day 28: Shine On

Find joy in the little things; they create the big picture.

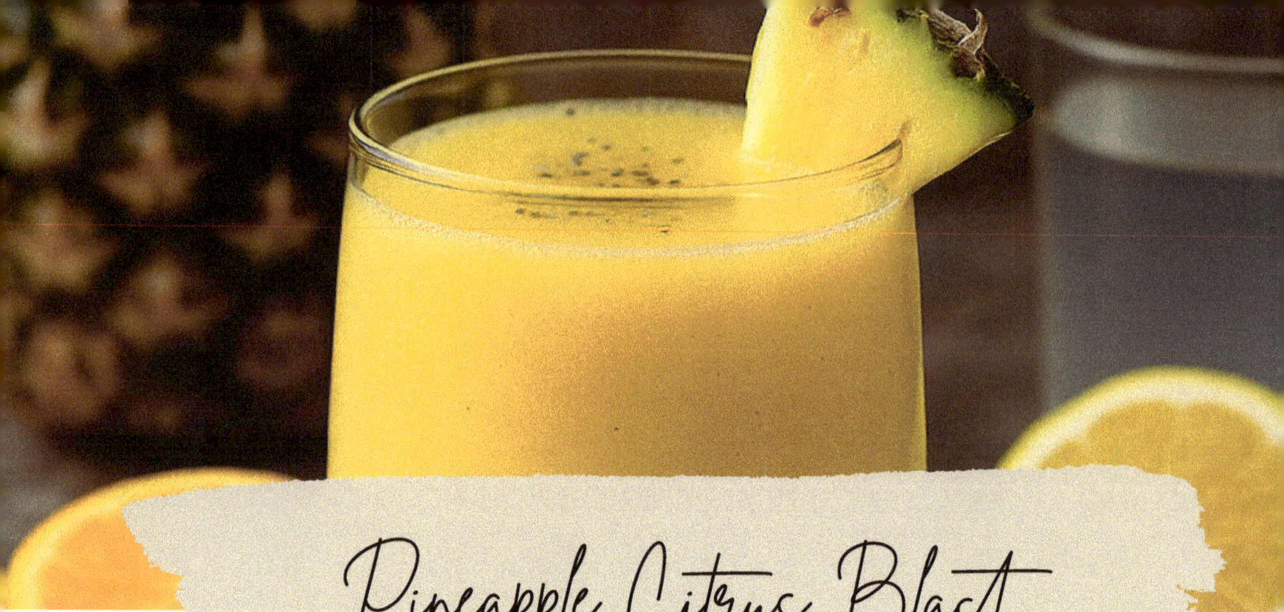

Pineapple Citrus Blast

Pineapple, orange, lemon, ginger, coconut water

The Pineapple Citrus Blast Smoothie is a vibrant and refreshing drink that combines the tropical sweetness of pineapple with the zesty brightness of orange and lemon, complemented by a zing of ginger. This uplifting smoothie is perfect for energizing your day and boosting your mood while providing essential hydration with coconut water.

INGREDIENTS:

- 1 cup fresh pineapple chunks
- 1 medium orange, peeled and segmented
- Juice of 1 lemon
- 1-inch piece of fresh ginger, peeled and grated
- 1 cup coconut water

OPTIONAL ADD-INS:

- 1 tablespoon chia seeds or flaxseeds: For added fiber and omega-3 fatty acids.
- 1 tbsp honey or agave syrup: If you desire additional sweetness.
- A handful of spinach: For extra nutrients without significantly altering the flavor.
- Ice cubes: For a colder, refreshing smoothie.

INSTRUCTIONS:

1. Peel and chop the pineapple into chunks if using fresh pineapple. Peel the orange and separate it into segments, removing any seeds as you go. Cut the lemon in half and squeeze out the juice, discarding any seeds. Peel and grate the ginger for easy blending.

2. In a high-speed blender, add the pineapple chunks, orange segments, lemon juice, grated ginger, and coconut water. If you're using optional ingredients, such as chia seeds, honey, or ice cubes, add them now. Blend on high until everything is smooth and creamy, about 30-60 seconds. Stop to scrape down the sides if necessary to ensure all ingredients are well combined. If the smoothie is too thick, you can thin it out by adding a small amount of coconut water.

3. Taste your Pineapple Citrus Blast Smoothie. If you want it sweeter, add more honey or agave syrup and blend again. Adjust the ginger or lime flavor if desired by adding more and mixing again. Pour the smoothie into a glass or a to-go container. For added flair, you can garnish with a slice of pineapple, a mint leaf, or a slice of orange. Enjoy immediately for maximum freshness and nutritional benefits!

TIPS:

- This smoothie is an excellent choice for a refreshing breakfast or an energizing snack throughout the day.
- You can experiment with other citrus fruits or tropical flavors, like lime or mango, for a unique twist.
- Prepare your ingredients in the evening for a quick and easy breakfast option the next day.

> *Enjoy your uplifting and refreshing Pineapple Citrus Blast Smoothie!*

“

Day 28: Shine On

I am a divine original.
Radiant. Whole. Free.

”

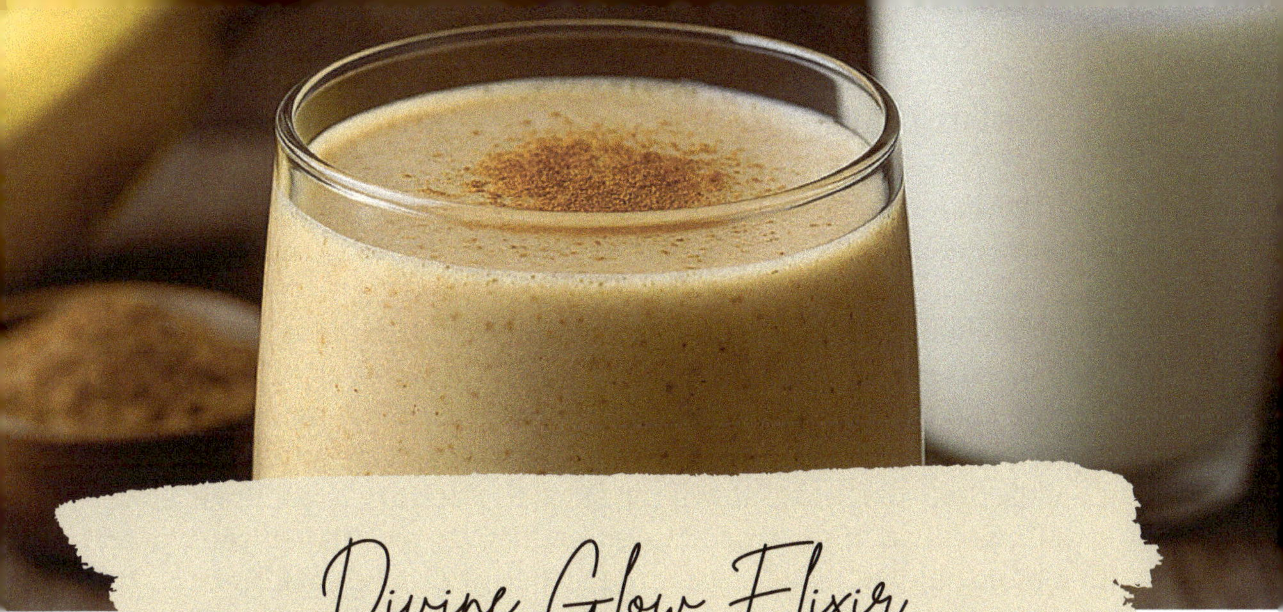

Divine Glow Elixir

Almond milk, banana, flax, vanilla, cinnamon

The Divine Glow Elixir Smoothie is a nourishing and celebratory blend that combines nourishing almond milk with the natural sweetness of banana, the nutritional power of flaxseed, and the comforting flavors of vanilla and cinnamon. This smoothie is designed to promote beauty from within, restore balance, and create a sense of peace, making it perfect for enjoying as part of your self-care routine or as a delightful treat at any time of day.

INGREDIENTS:

- 1 cup unsweetened almond milk
- 1 medium ripe banana
- 2 tablespoons ground flaxseed
- 1/2 teaspoon vanilla extract
- 1/2 teaspoon ground cinnamon

OPTIONAL ADD-INS:

- 1 tablespoon honey or maple syrup: For added sweetness, if desired.
- A pinch of sea salt: To enhance flavors and balance sweetness. - 1 tablespoon almond butter: For extra creaminess and healthy fats.
- Ice cubes: For a chilled smoothie.

INSTRUCTIONS:

1. Peel the banana and break it into chunks for more effortless blending. Measure out the almond milk, flaxseed, vanilla extract, and cinnamon.

2. In a high-speed blender, add the almond milk, banana, ground flaxseed, vanilla extract, and ground cinnamon. If you're using any optional ingredients, such as honey, almond butter, or ice cubes, add them now. Blend on high speed until the mixture is smooth and creamy, about 30 to 60 seconds. Stop and scrape down the sides if necessary to ensure everything is well combined. If the smoothie is too thick for your liking, you can add a little more almond milk or water to reach your desired consistency.

3. Taste your Divine Glow Elixir Smoothie. If you'd like it sweeter, add more honey or maple syrup and blend again. Adjust the amount of cinnamon or flaxseed to suit your taste preferences. Pour the smoothie into a glass or a to-go container. For an aesthetic touch, you can sprinkle a little extra cinnamon on top or garnish with a banana slice. Enjoy immediately to savor its fresh flavors and health benefits!

TIPS:

- This smoothie is perfect for a nourishing breakfast or a delightful snack that promotes beauty and balance.

- Consider preparing the ingredients ahead of time for a quick and easy smoothie in the morning.

- You can add other fruits, such as berries or tropical fruits, for additional flavors and benefits.

> *Enjoy your delicious and nourishing Divine Glow Elixir Smoothie as a celebration of beauty, balance, and peace!*

What does wellness mean to you today?

Radiate & *Glow Check-In*

> *Confidence, light, joy, wholeness.*

How has this journey changed how I see myself? What parts of me are now glowing that once felt hidden? What will I carry forward as I continue to prioritize my wellness, my joy, and my divine light?

Appendix

Recommended Equipment:

Blenders (Breville Super Q, Vitamix 5200, NutriBullet Pro, Ninja BL60)

Juicers (EanOruus, Nama J2, Ninja NeverClog, Kuvings AUTO10)

Other Tools: mesh strainer, mason jars, glass bottles, reusable produce bags

Storage and Prep Tools:

Mesh strainer, mason jars, glass bottles, reusable produce bags

Ice cube trays (for freezing extra juice or smoothie ingredients like ginger, lemon juice, or greens)

Meal prep containers (BPA-free glass or stackable containers for weekly ingredients)

Cutting board & sharp knife (high-quality prep tools make a big difference)

Citrus juicer or hand reamer (for fresh lemon and lime juice with ease)

Superfood boosters:

- Chia seeds, flaxseed, hemp hearts
- Maca powder, spirulina, collagen peptides

Protein powders:

- Plant-based (pea, hemp, or rice protein)
- Clean whey or collagen for added support

Suggested Pantry Staples

- Raw honey or maple syrup (natural sweeteners)
- Almond butter, peanut butter, or cashew butter
- Coconut water, almond milk, oat milk
- Apple cider vinegar (for shots or liver support)

Wellness Enhancers

- **Notebook** (for tracking how you feel, logging favorites)
- **Water bottle** (infuser bottles for lemon/mint water throughout the day)
- **Thermal smoothie cup** (to take smoothies on the go while keeping them fresh)

Apps & Digital Support

- Juice/smoothie ingredient tracker or habit tracker app
- Meditation or journaling apps (like Insight Timer or Day One)
- Barcode scanner app for checking additives in store-bought ingredients

The Power *in Every Pour*

Every ingredient has a purpose. Every blend is an act of love.

The ingredients in your smoothies aren't just fruits and greens—they're nature's medicine, created to support your healing, balance your body, and restore your glow from the inside out.

This is nourishment with intention.

This is food as fuel, as beauty, as energy, and as grace.

As you move through the next 28 days, you'll meet a variety of vibrant ingredients—each one selected to support your divine wellness journey. From hormone-balancing berries to bloat-busting ginger, these gifts from the earth are here to help you reclaim your body and feel good in your skin again.

Below, you'll find a list of key ingredients and the benefits they offer—so you can sip with even more clarity, confidence, and connection to your why.

This isn't just a smoothie.

It's a declaration. A reset. A return to yourself.

Let's meet the ingredients that are showing up for you—just like you're showing up for you.

Ingredient	Nutritional Benefit
Almond Butter	*Rich in healthy fats and protein, it supports satiety and helps maintain stable blood sugar levels.*
Almond Milk	*Low-calorie, dairy-free base rich in vitamin E for skin health.*
Aloe Juice	*It soothes the digestive tract and hydrates the body from within.*
Apple	*High in fiber and vitamin C, it supports healthy digestion and a strong immune system.*
Apple Cider Vinegar (ACV)	*It helps balance blood sugar and supports gut health.*
Ashwagandha	*An adaptogen that helps reduce stress and support hormonal balance.*
Avocado	*Loaded with heart-healthy fats, fiber, and skin-nourishing nutrients.*
Banana	*It provides potassium, natural sweetness, and a smooth texture.*
Beet	*It boosts blood flow, supports liver detox, and enhances stamina.*
Blueberries	*Antioxidant-rich; promotes brain, heart, and skin health.*
Cacao Powder	*Mood-boosting and high in magnesium and antioxidants.*
Carrot	*Packed with beta-carotene for skin and eye health.*
Cashew Butter	*Creamy source of healthy fats and magnesium.*
Celery	*Hydrating helps reduce inflammation.*
Chamomile Tea	*It calms the nervous system and promotes restful sleep.*
Chia Seeds	*High in omega-3s and fiber, this supports digestion and promotes fullness.*
Cinnamon	*It regulates blood sugar and adds natural warmth to blends.*
Clementines	*Similar to oranges, it is high in vitamin C and refreshing.*
Coconut Milk	*It adds creaminess and healthy fats, making it an excellent choice for boosting energy.*

Coconut Water	*Hydrating and full of electrolytes.*
Cold Brew Coffee	*Natural energy boost and antioxidant support.*
Cucumber	*Hydrating and soothing to the digestive tract.*
Dates	*It is a natural sweetener with fiber and trace minerals.*
Flaxseed	*Supports hormonal balance and gut health with omega-3 fatty acids and fiber.*
Ginger	*Reduces inflammation and soothes the digestive system.*
Green Apple	*Crisp, tangy, and high in fiber and antioxidants.*
Honey	*It is a natural sweetener with antibacterial properties and trace minerals.*
Honeydew Melon	*Hydrating and rich in vitamin C.*
Kale	*Nutrient-dense leafy green loaded with antioxidants, fiber, and calcium.*
Lemon	*It is alkalizing and high in vitamin C, supporting immunity and promoting a radiant skin glow.*
Lime	*Brightens flavor and supports detox with vitamin C.*
Maca Powder	*It boosts energy and supports hormonal balance.*
Mango	*Rich in enzymes and vitamins A and C, it promotes healthy digestion and skin.*
Melon (General)	*Hydrating and refreshing, full of vitamins and water.*
Mint	*It cools the body, freshens breath, and soothes digestion.*
Mixed Berries	*Antioxidant-packed blend that supports heart and skin health.*
Nutmeg	*It adds warmth and supports digestion.*
Oat Milk	*The smooth, dairy-free base supports satiety and is easy on digestion.*
Orange	*Immunity-boosting and brightens mood with vitamin C.*

Papaya	*Rich in enzymes (papain) for gut health and skin vibrance.*
Peach	*Juicy and vitamin-rich; supports hydration and digestion.*
Peanut Butter	*Protein-rich and satisfying; great for energy.*
Pear	*It is high in fiber and gentle on the digestive system.*
Pineapple	*It contains bromelain to ease digestion and reduce inflammation.*
Plum	*Gentle laxative effect; supports regularity and antioxidants.*
Power Greens	*A blend of kale, spinach, and other dark leafy greens—nutrient-packed.*
Pumpkin Purée	*Rich in fiber and beta-carotene for hormone and gut support.*
Spinach	*Mild green is rich in iron, folate, and antioxidants.*
Strawberries	*It is rich in vitamin C and antioxidants, supporting skin and heart health.*
Tahini	*Ground sesame seed paste is rich in calcium and healthy fats.*
Tangerines	*Sweet citrus option rich in vitamin C.*
Turmeric	*Powerful anti-inflammatory and antioxidant.*

Nourish Beyond *the Blend*

Because wellness doesn't stop at the glass.

You've just completed a soul-centered, smoothie-powered reset—and now, your body is craving continued nourishment that feels just as intentional.

This next chapter isn't about going back to old habits. It's about building a new rhythm—one where meals are just as healing, grounding, and grace-filled as the smoothies you've come to love.

This is your invitation to carry that same energy—of mindfulness, presence, and divine care—into your everyday meals and snacks. The recipes that follow are simple, delicious, and designed to **support your glow, gut, and goals** long after your 28 days.

Let them serve as inspiration—not instruction. Add your flavors. Trust your body. Stay rooted in what feels good.
This is nourishment on your terms.

Because still—**it's your turn.**

Enjoy a few of *my favorite meals*

A continuation of divine nourishment beyond your smoothie journey

Quinoa Power Bowl
Ingredients: Quinoa, roasted sweet potato, sautéed kale, avocado, chickpeas, tahini drizzle
Why it works: Balanced, plant-powered, hormone-supportive

Salmon + Garlic Greens
Ingredients: Baked salmon, sautéed spinach or broccoli, garlic, olive oil, lemon
Why it works: Omega-3s, detox-friendly, anti-inflammatory

Turkey Lettuce Wraps
Ingredients: Ground turkey, shredded carrots, scallions, coconut aminos, romaine leaves
Why it works: Light, low-carb, protein-rich and satisfying

Chickpea Curry Bowl
Ingredients: Chickpeas, coconut milk, turmeric, spinach, garlic, cumin, brown rice
Why it works: Plant-based, fiber-rich, supports hormone detox

Sweet Potato & Black Bean Tacos
Ingredients: Roasted sweet potatoes, black beans, avocado, red cabbage, lime crema
Why it works: High in fiber, anti-inflammatory, energizing

Grilled Shrimp & Avocado Salad
Ingredients: Mixed greens, grilled shrimp, avocado, cucumber, lemon vinaigrette
Why it works: Light, refreshing, supports skin and digestion.

Glow-Up Stir Fry
Ingredients: Broccoli, bell peppers, mushrooms, garlic, tofu or chicken, sesame oil
Why it works: Easy, colorful, nutrient-dense and energizing

Mediterranean Bowl
Ingredients: Hummus, quinoa, cherry tomatoes, cucumber, olives, roasted chickpeas
Why it works: Balanced, rich in healthy fats and plant protein

Warm Lentil + Veggie Soup
Ingredients: Green lentils, carrots, celery, kale, herbs, veggie broth
Why it works: Warming, high fiber, gut-healing

Baked Lemon Herb Cod + Roasted Veggies
Ingredients: Cod fillet, lemon, garlic, roasted zucchini, squash, and carrots
Why it works: Light protein, easy digestion, skin-brightening

Stuffed Bell Peppers
Ingredients: Bell peppers filled with quinoa, black beans, onions, tomatoes, and herbs
Why it works: Great for batch cooking, satisfying and hormone-supportive

Spaghetti Squash Pasta
Ingredients: Roasted spaghetti squash, cherry tomatoes, garlic, olive oil, basil, optional feta
Why it works: Low-carb, anti-inflammatory, deliciously light

Wild Rice + Mushroom Bowl
Ingredients: Wild rice, sautéed mushrooms, garlic, kale, drizzle of truffle or olive oil
Why it works: Earthy, grounding, rich in B vitamins for mood support

Zucchini Noodles + Pesto Chicken
Ingredients: Spiralized zucchini, grilled chicken, homemade basil pesto
Why it works: Clean, protein-rich, and beautifully anti-inflammatory

Why the Sunflower...

One of my favorite flowers

A symbol of light, strength, and sacred return

The sunflower is more than a beautiful bloom—it is a symbol of unwavering strength, spiritual alignment, and radiant joy. With its golden petals reaching for the sun, it naturally turns its face toward light, even on cloudy days. This instinct to seek light is what makes the sunflower such a powerful metaphor for wellness and self-reclamation.

The sunflower reminds us that healing is not about becoming someone new, but about returning to the vibrant, whole version of ourselves that was always there. Like the sunflower, we are divinely designed to grow—even in imperfect soil—and to rise with grace, regardless of the shadows that surround us.

The sunflower is also a symbol of consistency and devotion to self. It reflects the daily decision to show up, to nourish your body, to protect your peace, and to align your life with purpose and light.

You are a divine original—rooted in purpose, blooming in your own season, and rising toward your own light. This journey is not just a reset—it's a radiant return to YOU.

Let the sunflower be your reminder:
To turn toward what nourishes you
To bloom boldly, unapologetically
To rise, again and again

This is your time. This is your turn.

A Divine *Send-Off*

You came here for a reset. But what you did was so much more.

You showed up—for your body, your energy, your voice, your breath. You blended intention into every glass, and you poured presence into every page. This wasn't just a 28-day plan. It was a sacred return. A reset, yes. But also, a reclamation. A recharge.

A remembering of who you've always been.

And that divine original? She's still unfolding.

As this chapter closes, the journey continues—not with pressure, but with possibility. Continue to nourish yourself with what feels right. Keep pausing. Keep journaling. Your journal is your mirror, your altar, your companion in truth. Let it be the place where you release, realign, and rise.

Let it be the place where you keep reclaiming your time. Your energy. Your purpose.

Because it's still your turn, every day, you wake up and choose yourself again, it's your turn.

And now, a parting poem for the divine original you are and always will be

"Turn Toward the Light: It's My Turn"
by Tarsha W. Calloway

I gave, I moved, I made space for the world—
Until one day, I looked inward and saw a girl.
Who had waited in silence, waited in grace,
To take up her rhythm, reclaim her place.
With every blend, I remembered my name.
With every sip, I softened the shame.
With every word, I wrote myself whole—
This is the journey that nourished my soul.
Not for shrinking but for light.
Not to be perfect, but to feel right.
This is not the end, just the rise—
Of a woman who dares to prioritize.
She is bold. She is true.
She is healing, becoming, breaking through.
This is her season. Her healing. Her climb.

This is her whisper:
"It's my turn."

Keep Writing *Keep Blooming...*

This is not the end of your journey—this is the beginning of a deeper, more sacred return to yourself.

As you move forward beyond these 28 days, let these pages be your space to continue listening inward, dreaming boldly, and choosing you. Journaling is a gift you give yourself—an invitation to release, to remember, and to reconnect.

Write when you're celebrating.
Write when you're healing.
Write when you're unsure but still choosing to grow.

Your thoughts are seeds. Your words, water.
And this space? It's where you continue to bloom.

Because you are a divine original, and your story is still unfolding.
Keep writing, keep reclaiming.
It's still your turn.

What has this journey awakened in me?
What truths have I remembered?
What habits, emotions, or limiting beliefs am I ready to release?
What do I now understand about who I am, what I need, and how I want to feel—every single day?

How will I continue to reclaim my time, protect my peace, and nourish my body, mind, and spirit moving forward?

About the *Author*

Meet Tarsha W. Calloway—a proud mom, loving wife, loyal friend, nurturer, entrepreneur, and philanthropic leader. She committed to selflessly empowering others to become the best version of themselves. She is embarking on a transformative journey to reclaim her health, confirm her joy, and live in her purpose. This 28-day self-reflection and wellness guide stems from her decision to invite —parents, caretakers, and all whom she loves—to embrace simplicity, grace, and prioritize self-care.

Raised in a community that cherished family, and compassion and empathy, Tarsha knows the profound impact of small acts of kindness. Her innovative spirit and engaging presence have earned her recognition as a leader in philanthropy and social entrepreneurship, allowing her to address pressing community needs with creativity and love. Through this journey, Tarsha inspires everyone to step into their purpose by focusing on self, inner healing, and reclaiming their time. She encourages readers to honor their unique journeys and choose themselves, one intentional day at a time.

You are a divine original, beautifully equipped to bloom in your own time.

I am a Divine Original

Drink Beautifully. Feel Divine

www.ingramcontent.com/pod-product-compliance
Lightning Source LLC
LaVergne TN
LVHW070908210926
848482LV00017B/1025